[redacted]

3rd Edition

Psych Notes

Clinical Pocket Guide

Darlene D. Pedersen, MSN, APRN, PMHCNS

Pur your
hea)avis
by r by
call N)

A Davis's Notes Book

F.A. Davis Company • Philadelphia

F. A. Davis Company
1915 Arch Street
Philadelphia, PA 19103
www.fadavis.com

Printed in China

Last digit indicates print number: 10 9 8 7 6 5 4 3 2

Publisher, Nursing: Robert G. Martone
Sr. Developmental Editor: William F. Welsh
Sr. Project Editor: Padraic J. Maroney
Manager of Art & Design: Carolyn O'Brien
Reviewers: Peggy Bozarth, MSN, RN, CNE, Sherry Campbell, MS, APRN, PMH, BC, CNE Bonnie Clark, RN, MSN-ED, FNP, Martha M. Colvin, Ph.D., RN, Jacqueline Kern, PhD, RN, ACHPN, Brenda G. Kucirka, PhD(c) RN, PMHCNS-BC, CNE, Ramel F. Moore, PMHCNS-BC , Dana Olive, PhD, CRNP, Karen A. Peterson, RN, PMHCNS, BC, Theresa Pietsch, PhD, RN, Colleen M. Quinn, RN, MSN, EdD,(c), Patti Scott, RN, MSN, ARNP-FNP, Jan S. Watts, RN, MSN, Roberta Weseman, MSN, RN, Jeana Wilcox, PhD, RN, CNS, CNE , Debra Rose Wilson, PhD, MSN, RN, IBCLC, AHN-BC, CHT.

Place 2⅞ × 2⅞ **Sticky Notes** here
for a convenient and refillable note pad

✓**HIPAA compliant**
✓**OSHA compliant**

Waterproof and Reusable
Wipe-Free Pages

Write directly onto any page of
Psych Notes: Clinical Pocket Guide
with a ballpoint pen. Wipe old entries
off with an alcohol pad and reuse.

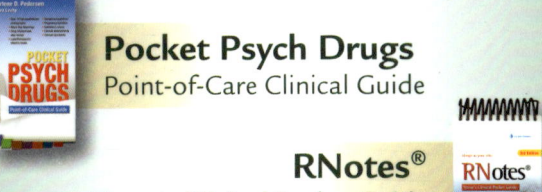

Mental Health and Mental Illness: Basics

Mental Health and Mental Illness: Basics

Mental health and mental illness have been defined in many ways but should always be viewed in the context of ethnocultural factors and influence.

Mental Illness/Disorder

The DSM-IV-TR defines mental illness/disorder (paraphrased) as: *a clinically significant behavioral or psychological syndrome or pattern associated with distress or disability...with increased risk of death, pain, disability and is not a reasonable (expectable) response to a particular situation (APA 2000).* The DSM-5 is slated to publish in May of 2013.

Mental Health

Mental health is defined as: *a state of successful performance of mental function, resulting in productive activities, fulfilling relationships with other people, and the ability to adapt to change and cope with adversity (US Surgeon General Report, Dec 1999).*

Wellness-illness continuum – Dunn's 1961 text, *High Level Wellness,* altered our concept of health and illness, viewing both as on a continuum that was dynamic and changing, focusing on *levels of wellness.* Concepts include: totality, uniqueness, energy, self-integration, energy use, and inner/outer worlds.

Legal Definition of Mental Illness

The legal definition of insanity/mental illness applies the M'Naghten Rule, formulated in 1843 and derived from English law. It says that: *a person is innocent by reason of insanity if at the time of committing the act, [the person] was laboring under a defect of reason from disease of the mind as not to know the nature and quality of the act being done, or if he did know it, he did not know that what he was doing was wrong.* There are variations of this legal definition by state, and some states have abolished the insanity defense.

Positive Mental Health: Jahoda's Six Major Categories

In 1958, Marie Jahoda developed six major categories of positive mental health:

- Attitudes of individual toward self
- Presence of growth and development, or actualization
- Personality integration

- Autonomy and independence
- Perception of reality, and
- Environmental mastery

The mentally healthy person accepts the self, is self-reliant, and is self-confident.

Maslow's Hierarchy of Needs

Maslow developed a hierarchy of needs based on attainment of self-actualization, where one becomes highly evolved and attains his or her full potential.

The basic belief is that lower-level needs must be met first in order to advance to the next level of needs. Therefore, physiological and safety needs must be met before issues related to love and belonging can be addressed, through to self-actualization.

Maslow's Hierarchy of Needs	
Self-Actualization	Self-fulfillment/reach highest potential
Self-Esteem	Seek self-respect, achieve recognition
Love/Belonging	Giving/receiving affection, companionship
Safety and Security	Avoiding harm; order, structure, protection
Physiological	Air, water, food, shelter, sleep, elimination

General Adaptation Syndrome (Stress-Adaptation Syndrome)

Hans Selye (1976) divided his *stress syndrome* into three stages and, in doing so, pointed out the seriousness of prolonged stress on the body and the need for identification and intervention.

1. **Alarm stage** – This is the immediate physiological (fight or flight) response to a threat or perceived threat.
2. **Resistance** – If the stress continues, the body adapts to the levels of stress and attempts to return to homeostasis.
3. **Exhaustion** – With prolonged exposure and adaptation, the body eventually becomes depleted. There are no more reserves to draw upon, and serious illness may now develop (e.g., hypertension, mental disorders, cancer). Selye teaches us that without intervention, even death is a possibility at this stage.

CLINICAL PEARL: *Identification and treatment* of chronic, posttraumatic stress disorder (PTSD) and unresolved grief, including multiple (compounding) losses, are critical in an attempt to prevent serious illness and improve quality of life.

Fight-or-Flight Response

In the fight-or-flight response, if a person is presented with a stressful situation (danger), a physiological response (sympathetic nervous system) activates the adrenal glands and cardiovascular system, allowing a person to rapidly adjust to the need to fight or flee a situation.

- Such physiological response is beneficial in the short term: for instance, in an emergency situation.
- However, with ongoing, chronic psychological stressors, a person continues to experience the same physiological response as if there were a real danger, which eventually physically and emotionally depletes the body.

Diathesis-Stress Model

The diathesis-stress model views behavior as the result of *genetic* and *biological factors*. A genetic predisposition results in a mental disorder (e.g., mood disorder or schizophrenia) when precipitated by environmental factors.

Theories of Personality Development

Psychoanalytic Theory

Sigmund Freud, who introduced us to the Oedipus complex, hysteria, free association, and dream interpretation, is considered the "Father of Psychiatry." He was concerned with both the dynamics and structure of the psyche. He divided the personality into three parts:

- **Id** – The id developed out of Freud's concept of the pleasure principle. The id comprises primitive, instinctual drives (hunger, sex, aggression). The id says, "I want."
- **Ego** – It is the ego, or rational mind, that is called upon to control the instinctual impulses of the self-indulgent id. The ego says, "I think/I evaluate."
- **Superego** – The superego is the conscience of the psyche and monitors the ego. The superego says "I should/I ought" (Hunt 1994).

Topographic Model of the Mind

Freud's topographic model deals with levels of awareness and is divided into three categories:

- **Unconscious mind** – All mental content and memories *outside of conscious awareness;* becomes conscious through the preconscious mind.
- **Preconscious mind** – Not within the conscious mind but *can more easily be brought to conscious awareness* (repressive function of instinctual desires or undesirable memories). Reaches consciousness through word linkage.
- **Conscious mind** – All content and memories *immediately available and within conscious awareness.* Of lesser importance to psychoanalysts.

Key Defense Mechanisms	
Defense Mechanism	**Example**
Denial – Refuses to accept a painful reality, pretending as if it doesn't exist.	A man who snorts cocaine daily, is fired for attendance problems, yet insists he doesn't have a problem.
Displacement – Directing anger toward someone or onto another, less threatening (safer) substitute.	An older employee is publicly embarrassed by a younger boss at work and angrily cuts a driver off on the way home.
Identification – Taking on attributes and characteristics of someone admired.	A young man joins the police academy to become a policeman like his father, whom he respects.
Intellectualization – Excessive focus on logic and reason to avoid the feelings associated with a situation.	An executive who has cancer requests all studies and blood work and discusses in detail with her doctor, as if she were speaking about someone else.
Projection – Attributing to others feelings unacceptable to self.	A group therapy client strongly dislikes another member but claims that it is the member who "dislikes her."
Reaction Formation – Expressing an opposite feeling from what is actually felt and is considered undesirable.	John, who despises Jeremy, greets him warmly and offers him food and beverages and special attention.

Continued

Key Defense Mechanisms—cont'd

Defense Mechanism	Example
Sublimation – Redirecting unacceptable feelings or drives into an acceptable channel.	A mother of a child killed in a drive-by shooting becomes involved in legislative change for gun laws and gun violence.
Undoing – Ritualistically negating or undoing intolerable feelings/thoughts.	A man who has thoughts that his father will die must step on sidewalk cracks to prevent this and cannot miss a crack.

Stages of Personality Development

Freud's Psychosexual Development

Age	Stage	Task
0–18 mo	Oral	Oral gratification
18 mo–3 yr	Anal	Independence and control (voluntary sphincter control)
3–6 yr	Phallic	Genital focus
6–12 yr	Latency	Repressed sexuality; channeled sexual drives (sports)
13–20 yr	Genital	Puberty with sexual interest in opposite sex

Sullivan's Interpersonal Theory

Age	Stage	Task
0–18 mo	Infancy	Anxiety reduction via oral gratification
18 mo–6 yr	Childhood	Delay in gratification

Continued

Sullivan's Interpersonal Theory—cont'd

Age	Stage	Task
6–9 yr	Juvenile	Satisfying peer relationships
9–12 yr	Preadolescence	Satisfying same-sex relationships
12–14 yr	Early adolescence	Satisfying opposite-sex relationships
14–21 yr	Late adolescence	Lasting intimate opposite-sex relationship

Erikson's Psychosocial Theory

Age	Stage	Task
0–18 mo	Trust vs. mistrust	Basic trust in mother figure and generalizes
18 mo–3 yr	Autonomy vs. shame/doubt	Self-control/independence
3–6 yr	Initiative vs. guilt	Initiate and direct own activities
6–12 yr	Industry vs. inferiority	Self-confidence through successful performance and recognition
12–20 yr	Identity vs. role confusion	Task integration from previous stages; secure sense of self
20–30 yr	Intimacy vs. isolation	Form a lasting relationship or commitment
30–65 yr	Generativity vs. stagnation	Achieve life's goals; consider future generations
65 yr–death	Ego integrity vs. despair	Life review with meaning from both positives and negatives; positive self-worth

Mahler's Theory of Object Relations

Age	Phase (subphase)	Task
0–1 mo	1. Normal autism	Basic needs fulfillment (for survival)
1–5 mo	2. Symbiosis 3. Separation – individuation	Awareness of external fulfillment source
5–10 mo	– *Differentiation*	Commencement of separateness from mother figure
10–16 mo	– *Practicing*	Locomotor independence; awareness of separateness of self
16–24 mo	– *Rapprochement*	Acute separateness awareness; seeks emotional refueling from mother figure
24–36 mo	– *Consolidation*	Established sense of separateness; internalizes sustained image of loved person/object when out of sight; separation anxiety resolution

Peplau's Interpersonal Theory

Age	Stage	Task
Infant	Depending on others	Learning ways to communicate with primary caregiver for meeting comfort needs
Toddler	Delaying satisfaction	Some delay in self-gratification to please others
Early Childhood	Self-identification	Acquisition of appropriate roles and behaviors through perception of others' expectations of self
Late Childhood	Participation skills	Competition, compromise, cooperation skills acquisition; sense of one's place in the world

Stages of Personality Development tables modified from Townsend MC. Essentials of Psychiatric Mental Health Nursing, 5th ed. Philadelphia: FA Davis, 2010, used with permission

Biological Aspects of Mental Illness

Mind-Body Dualism to Brain and Behavior

- René Descartes (17th C) espoused the theory of the mind-body dualism (Cartesian dualism), wherein the mind (soul) was said to be completely separate from the body.
- Current research and approaches show the connection between mind and body and that newer treatments will develop from a better understanding of both the biological and psychological (Hunt 1994).
- The US Congress stated that the 1990s would be "The Decade of the Brain," with increased focus and research in the areas of neurobiology, genetics, and biological markers.
- The Decade of Behavior (2000–2010) is a "multidisciplinary" initiative launched by the American Psychological Association (APA), focusing on the behavioral and social sciences, trying to address major challenges facing the US today in health, safety, education, prosperity, and democracy (www.decadeofbehavior.org).

Central and Peripheral Nervous System

Central Nervous System

- Brain
  - Forebrain:
    - *Cerebrum (frontal, parietal, temporal, and occipital lobes)*
    - *Diencephalon (thalamus, hypothalamus, and limbic system)*
  - Midbrain
    - *Mesencephalon*
  - Hindbrain
    - Pons, medulla, and cerebellum
- Nerve Tissue
  - Neurons
  - Synapses
  - Neurotransmitters
- Spinal Cord
  - Fiber tracts
  - Spinal nerves

Continued

Peripheral Nervous System

- Afferent System
  - Sensory neurons (somatic and visceral)
- Efferent System
  - Somatic nervous system (somatic motor neurons)
  - Autonomic nervous system
    - Sympathetic nervous system
      Visceral motor neurons
    - Parasympathetic nervous system
      Visceral motor neurons

The Brain

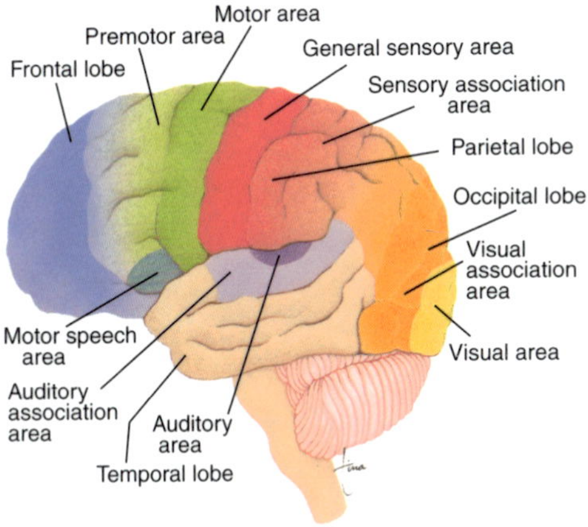

Left cerebral hemisphere showing some of the functional areas that have been mapped. (From Scanlon VC, Sanders T. Essentials of Anatomy and Physiology, 6th ed. FA Davis: Philadelphia, 2011, used with permission)

Limbic System

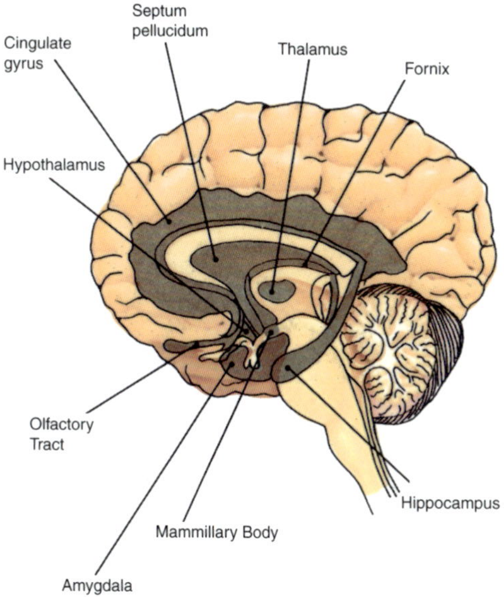

The limbic system and its structures. (Adapted from Scanlon VC, Sanders T. Essentials of Anatomy and Physiology, 6th ed. FA Davis: Philadelphia, 2011, used with permission)

Sympathetic and Parasympathetic Effects

Structure	Sympathetic	Parasympathetic
Eye (pupil)	Dilation	Constriction
Nasal Mucosa	Mucus reduction	Mucus increased
Salivary Gland	Saliva reduction	Saliva increased
Heart	Rate increased	Rate decreased
Arteries	Constriction	Dilation
Lung	Bronchial muscle relaxation	Bronchial muscle contraction
Gastrointestinal Tract	Decreased motility	Increased motility
Liver	Conversion of glycogen to glucose increased	Glycogen synthesis
Kidney	Decreased urine	Increased urine
Bladder	Contraction of sphincter	Relaxation of sphincter
Sweat Glands	↑ Sweating	No change

Synapse Transmission

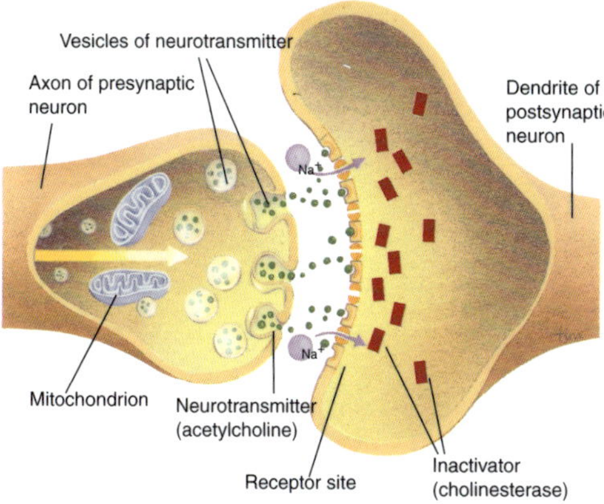

Impulse transmission at a synapse. Arrows indicate direction of electrical impulse. (From Scanlon VC, Sanders T. Essentials of Anatomy and Physiology, 6th ed. FA Davis: Philadelphia, 2011, used with permission)

Neurotransmitters

Neurotransmitter Functions and Effects

Neurotransmitter	Function	Effect
Dopamine	Inhibitory	Fine movement, emotional behavior. Implicated in schizophrenia and Parkinson's.
Serotonin	Inhibitory	Sleep, mood, eating behavior. Implicated in mood disorders, anxiety, and violence.

Continued

Neurotransmitter Functions and Effects—cont'd

Neurotransmitter	Function	Effect
Norepinephrine	Excitatory	Arousal, wakefulness, learning. Implicated in anxiety and addiction.
Gamma-aminobutyric acid (GABA)	Inhibitory	Anxiety states.
Acetylcholine	Excitatory	Arousal, attention, movement. Increase = spasms and decrease = paralysis.

Legal-Ethical Issues

Confidentiality

Confidentiality in all of health care is important but notably so in psychiatry because of possible discriminatory treatment of those with mental illness. All individuals have a right to privacy, and all client records and communications should be kept confidential.

Do's and Don'ts of Confidentiality

- Do not discuss clients by using their actual names or any identifier that could be linked to a particular client (e.g., name/date of birth on an x-ray/assessment form).
- Do not discuss client particulars outside of a private, professional environment. Do not discuss with family members or friends.
- Be particularly careful in elevators of hospitals or community centers. You never know who might be on the elevator with you.
- Even in educational presentations, protect client identity by changing names (John Doe) and obtaining all (informed consent) permissions.
- Every client has the right to confidential and respectful treatment.
- Accurate, objective record keeping is important, and documentation is significant legally in demonstrating what was actually done for client care. If not documented, treatments are not considered done.

When Confidentiality Must Be Breached

- ***Confidentiality and Child Abuse*** – If it is suspected or clear that a child is being abused or in danger of abuse (physical/sexual/emotional) or neglect, the health professional must report such abuse as mandated by the Child Abuse Prevention Treatment Act, originally enacted in 1974 (PL 93–247).
- ***Confidentiality and Elder Abuse*** – If suspected or clear that an elder is being abused or in danger of abuse or neglect, then the health professional must also report this abuse.

- ***Tarasoff Principle/Duty to Warn*** (*Tarasoff v. Regents* of the University of California 1976) – Refers to the responsibility of a therapist, health professional, or nurse to warn a potential victim of imminent danger (a threat to harm person) and breach confidentiality. **The person in danger and others (able to protect person) must be notified of the intended harm.**

The Health Insurance Portability and Accountability Act (HIPAA) (1996)

Enacted on August 21, 1996, HIPAA was established with the goal of assuring that an individual's health information is properly protected while allowing the flow of health information (US Department of Health and Human Services, 2006; HIPAA, 2006).

Types of Commitment

- **Voluntary** – An individual decides treatment is needed and admits himself/herself to a hospital, leaving of own volition – unless a professional (psychiatrist/other professional) decides that the person is a danger to himself/herself or others.
- **Involuntary** – Involuntary commitments include: 1) emergency commitments, including those unable to care for self (basic personal needs) and 2) involuntary outpatient commitment (IOC).
  - ***Emergency*** – Involves ***imminent*** danger to self or others; has demonstrated a ***clear and present danger to self or others.*** Usually initiated by health professionals, authorities, and sometimes friends or family. Person is threatening to harm self or others. Or evidence that the person is unable to care for herself or himself (nourishment, personal, medical, safety) with reasonable probability that death will result within a month.
  - ***302 Emergency Involuntary Commitment*** – If a person is an *immediate danger to self or others* or is *in danger due to a lack of ability to care for self,* then an emergency psychiatric evaluation may be filed (section 302). This person must then be evaluated by a psychiatrist and released, or psychiatrist may uphold petition (patient admitted for up to 5 days). (Emergency commitments 2004; Christy et al 2010)

Restraints and Seclusion for an Adult – Behavioral Health Care

The Joint Commission on Accreditation of Healthcare Organizations (JCAHO) wants to reduce the use of behavioral restraints but has set forth guidelines for safety in the event they are used.

- In an emergency situation, restraints may be applied by an authorized and qualified staff member, but an order must be obtained from a Licensed Independent Practitioner (LIP) within 1 hour of initiation of restraints/seclusion.
- Following application of restraints, the following time frames must be adhered to for reevaluation/reordering:

    - Within first hour, physician or LIP must evaluate the patient face to face, after initiation of restraint/seclusion, if hospital uses accreditation for Medicare-deemed status purposes. If not for deemed status, LIP performs face-to-face evaluation within 4 hours of initiation of restraint/seclusion.
    - If adult is released prior to expiration of original order, LIP must perform a face-to-face evaluation within 24 hours of initiation of restraint/seclusion.
    - LIP reorders restraint every 4 hours until adult is released from restraint/seclusion. A qualified RN or other authorized staff person reevaluates individual and need to continue restraint/seclusion.
    - LIP face-to-face evaluation every 8 hours until patient is released from restraint/seclusion.
    - 4-hour RN or other qualified staff reassessment and 8-hour face-to-face evaluation repeated, as long as restraint /seclusion clinically necessary (JCAHO revised 2005).
- The *American Psychiatric Nurses Association* and *International Society of Psychiatric-Mental Health Nurses* are committed to the *reduction of seclusion and restraint* and have developed position statements, with a vision of eventually eliminating seclusion and restraint (APNA 2007; ISPN 1999).
- Learn your institutional policies on restraints and seclusion and take advantage of any training available, contacting supervisors/managers if any questions about protocols.

ALERT: The decision to initiate seclusion or restraint is made only after all other less restrictive, nonphysical methods have failed to resolve the behavioral emergency (APNA 2001). Restraint of a patient may be both physical and pharmacological (chemical) and infringes on a patient's freedom of movement and may result in injury (physical or psychological) and/or death. There must be an evaluation based on benefit: risk consideration and a leaning toward alternative solutions. Restraints may be used when there is dangerous behavior and to protect the patient and others. You need to become familiar with the standards as set forth by JCAHO and any state regulations and hospital policies. *The least restrictive method should be used and considered first, before using more restrictive interventions.*

A Patient's Bill of Rights

- First adopted in 1973 by the American Hospital Association, A Patient's Bill of Rights was revised on October 21, 1992.
- Sets forth an expectation of treatment and care that will allow for improved collaboration between patients, health care providers, and institutions resulting in better patient care (American Hospital Association [revised] 1992).

The Patient Care Partnership

In 2003 "A Patient's Bill of Rights" was replaced by "The Patient Care Partnership," in order to emphasize the collaboration between patient and health providers (American Hospital Association 2003).

Quality and Safety Education for Nurses (QSEN)

The Quality and Safety Education for Nurses (QSEN) project (2005), funded by the Robert Wood Johnson Foundation, focused on the promotion of quality and safety in patient care. Teaching strategies include the following core competencies, which are needed to develop student and graduate attitudes and skills for quality patient care and safety: evidence-based practice, safety, teamwork and collaboration, patient-centered care, quality improvement and informatics (QSEN 2011). Additional information, including QSEN teaching strategies, can be found in Townsend: Essentials of Psychiatric Mental Health Nursing, 5th ed. (2010) and other resources.

Informed Consent

- Every adult person has the right to decide what can and cannot be done to his or her own body (*Schloendorff v. Society of New York Hospital,* 105 NE 92 [NY 1914]).
- Assumes a person is capable of making an informed decision about own health care.
- State regulations vary, but mental illness does not mean that a person is or should be assumed incapable of making decisions related to his or her own care.
- Patients have a right to:
  - Information about their treatment and any procedures to be performed.
  - Know the inherent risks and benefits.

Without this information (specific information, risks, and benefits) a person cannot make an informed decision. The above also holds true for those who might participate in research. Videocasts on informed consent can be accessed at: http://videocast.nih.org (National Institutes of Health, Informed Consent: The ideal and the reality, Session 5 November 9, 2005).

Right to Refuse Treatment/Medication

- Just as a person has the right to accept treatment, he or she also has the right to refuse treatment to the extent permitted by the law and to be informed of the medical consequences of his/her actions.
- In some emergency situations, a patient can be medicated or treated against his/her will, but state laws vary, and so it is imperative to become knowledgeable about applicable state laws (American Hospital Association [revised] 1992; American Hospital Association 2003).

Health Care Reform and Behavioral Health

On March 23, 2010 Barack Obama signed into law a comprehensive health care and reform legislation. Extensive information can be found at: http://mentalhealthcarereform.org. This site explains and summarizes the law, provides timelines for implementation, discusses health reform and parity, and provides excellent links to other relevant organizations. The American Psychiatric Association has approved a position statement entitled Principles for Health Care Reform for Psychiatry (2008). It is important to keep current as to mental health care reform, parity, and reform legislation as it affects mental health care in the years to come.

Psychiatric Assessment

Psychiatric History and Assessment Tool

Identifying/Demographic Information

Name ______________ Room No. ________________

Primary Care Provider: ________________________________

DOB _____________ Age________ Sex ___________

Race: ______________ Ethnicity: ___________________

Marital Status: __________ No. Marriages: ______________

If married/divorced/separated/widowed, how long? _____________

Occupation/School (grade): __________________________

Highest Education Level: ___________________________

Religious Affiliation: ______________________________

City of Residence: ________________________________

Name/Phone # of Significant Other: ___________________

Primary Language Spoken: ___________________________

Accompanied by: _________________________________

Admitted from: __________________________________

Previous Psychiatric Hospitalizations (#): ______________________

Chief Complaint (in patient's own words): ____________________

DSM-IV Diagnosis (previous/current): _______________________

Nursing Diagnosis: ________________________________

Notes:

Family Members/Significant Others Living in Home			
Name	Relationship	Age	Occupation/Grade

Family Members/Significant Others Not in Home			
Name	Relationship	Age	Occupation/Grade

Children		
Name	Age	Living at Home?

CLINICAL PEARL: Compare what the client says with what other family members, friends, or significant others say about situations or previous treatments. It is usually helpful to gather information from those who have observed/lived with the client and can provide *another valuable source/side of information.* The *reliability of the client* in recounting the past must be considered and should be noted.

Genogram—See *Disorders/Intervention Tab* for sample genogram and common genogram symbols.

Past Psychiatric Treatments/Medications

It is important to obtain a history of any previous psychiatric hospitalizations, the number of hospitalizations and dates, and to record all current/past psychotropic medications, as well as other medications the client may be taking. Ask the client what has worked in the past, and also what has *not worked,* for both treatments and medications.

Inpatient Treatment

Facility/Location	Dates From/To	Diagnosis	Treatments	Response(s)

Outpatient Treatments/Services

Psychiatrist/Therapist	Location	Diagnosis	Treatment	Response(s)

Psychotropic Medications (Previous Treatments)

Name	Dose/Dosages	Treatment Length	Response	Comments

Current Psychotropic Medications

Name	Dose/Dosages	Date Started	Response(s)	Serum Levels

Other Current Medications, Herbals, and OTC Medications

Name	Dose/ Dosages	Date Started	Response(s)	Comments

CLINICAL PEARL: It is important to ask about any herbals, OTC medications (e.g., pseudoephedrine), or nontraditional treatments as client may not think to mention these when questioned about current medications. *Important herbals include, but are not limited to:* St. John's wort, ephedra (ma huang), ginseng, kava kava, and yohimbe. These can interact with psychotropics or other medications or cause anxiety and/or drowsiness, as well as other adverse physiological reactions. Be sure to record and then report any additional or herbal medications to the psychiatrist, advanced practice nurse, psychiatric nurse, and professional team staff.

Medical History (*See Clinical Pearls for Italics*)

TPR:	BP:
Height:	Weight:

Cardiovascular (CV)

Does client have or ever had the following disorders/symptoms (include date):

Hypertension	Murmurs	Chest Pain (Angina)
Palpitations/ Tachycardia	Shortness of Breath	Ankle Edema/Congestive Heart Failure
Fainting/Syncope	Myocardial Infarction	High Cholesterol
Leg Pain (Claudication)	*Arrhythmias*	*Other CV Disease*
Heart Bypass	Angioplasty	Other CV surgery

CLINICAL PEARL: Heterocyclic antidepressants must be used with caution with *cardiovascular disease*. Tricyclic antidepressants (TCAs) may produce life-threatening *arrhythmias* and ECG changes.

Central Nervous System (CNS)		
Does client have or ever had the following disorders/symptoms (include date):		
Headache	Head Injury	Tremors
Dizziness/Vertigo	Loss of Consciousness (LOC); how long?	Stroke
Myasthenia Gravis	*Parkinson's Disease*	*Dementia*
Brain Tumor	*Seizure Disorder*	Multiple Sclerosis
TIAs	Other	Surgery

CLINICAL PEARL: Remember that *myasthenia gravis* is a contraindication to the use of antipsychotics; *tremors* could be due to a disease such as *Parkinson's* or could be a side effect of a psychotropic (lithium/antipsychotic). Sometimes the elderly may be diagnosed as having *dementia* when in fact they are depressed (pseudodementia). Use TCAs cautiously with *seizure disorders;* bupropion use contraindicated in seizure disorder.

Dermatological/Skin		
Does client have or ever had the following disorders/symptoms (include date):		
Psoriasis	*Hair Loss*	Itching
Rashes	*Acne*	Other/Surgeries

CLINICAL PEARL: Lithium can precipitate psoriasis or psoriatic arthritis in patients with a history of *psoriasis*, or the psoriasis may be new onset. *Acne* is also a possible reaction to lithium (new onset or exacerbation), and lithium may result in, although rarely, *hair loss (alopecia). Rashes* in patients on carbamazepine or lamotrigine may be a sign of a life-threatening mucocutaneous reaction, such as Stevens-Johnson syndrome (SJS). Discontinue medication/immediate medical attention needed.

Endocrinology/Metabolic

Does client have or ever had the following disorders/symptoms (include date):

Polydipsia	Polyuria	*Diabetes Type 1 or 2*
Hyperthyroidism	*Hypothyroidism*	Hirsutism
Polycystic Ovarian Syndrome	Other	Surgery

CLINICAL PEARL: Clients on lithium should be observed and tested for *hypothyroidism*. Atypical and older antipsychotics are associated with *treatment-emergent diabetes (need periodic testing: FBS, HgbA1c, lipids; BMI, etc)*.

Eye, Ears, Nose, Throat

Does client have or ever had the following disorders/symptoms (include date):

Eye Pain	*Halo around Light Source*	*Blurring*
Red Eye	Double vision	Flashing Lights/ Floaters
Glaucoma	Tinnitus	Ear Pain/Otitis Media
Hoarseness	Other	Other/Surgery

CLINICAL PEARL: *Eye pain and halo around a light source* are possible symptoms of glaucoma. *Closed-angle glaucoma* is a true emergency and requires immediate medical attention to prevent blindness. Anticholinergics (low-potency antipsychotics [chlorpromazine] or tricyclics) can cause *blurred vision*. Check for *history of glaucoma* as antipsychotics are contraindicated.

Gastrointestinal

Does client have or ever had the following disorders/symptoms (include date):

Nausea & Vomiting	Diarrhea	*Constipation*
GERD	Crohn's Disease	Colitis
Colon Cancer	Irritable Bowel Syndrome	Other/Surgery

CLINICAL PEARL: *Nausea* is a common side effect of many medications; tricyclic antidepressants can cause *constipation*. Nausea seems to be more common with paroxetine. Over time clients may adjust to these side effects, therefore no decision should be made about effectiveness/side effects or changing medications without a reasonable trial.

Genitourinary/Reproductive

Does client have or ever had the following disorders/symptoms (include date):

Miscarriages? Y/N # When?		Abortions? Y/N # When?
Nipple Discharge	*Amenorrhea*	*Gynecomastia*
Lactation	Dysuria	Urinary Incontinence
Pregnancy Problems	*Postpartum Depression*	Sexual Dysfunction
Prostate Problems (BPH)	Menopause	Fibrocystic Breast Disease
Penile Discharge	UTI	Pelvic Pain
Renal Disease	Urinary Cancer	Breast Cancer
Other/Surgery Cancer	Other Gynecological	Other

CLINICAL PEARL: Antipsychotics have an effect on the endocrinological system by affecting the tuberoinfundibular system. Those on antipsychotics may experience *gynecomastia and lactation (men also)*. Women may experience *amenorrhea*. Some drugs (TCAs), such as amitriptyline, must be used with caution with *BPH*. *Postpartum depression* requires evaluation and treatment (*see Postpartum Major Depressive Episode in Disorders-Interventions Tab*). **Men should also be observed/evaluated for postpartum depression.**

Respiratory

Does client have or ever had (include date):

Chronic Cough	Sore Throat	Bronchitis
Asthma	COPD	Pneumonia
Cancer (Lung/Throat)	Sleep Apnea	Other/Surgery

Other Questions:

Allergies (food/environmental/pet/contact)

____

Diet ______________________________

Drug Allergies ______________________________

Accidents ______________________________

High Prolonged Fever ______________________________

Tobacco Use ______________________________

Childhood Illnesses ______________________________

Fractures ______________________________

Menses Began ______________________________

Birth Control ______________________________

Disabilities (hearing/speech/movement) ______________________________

Pain (describe/location/length of time [over or under 3 months]/severity between 1 [least] and 10 [worst])/Treatment

____

Family History

Mental Illness ______________________________

____

Medical Disorders ______________________________

____

Substance Abuse ______________________________

Please note who in the family has the problem/disorder.

Substance Use

Prescribed Drugs

Name	Dosage	Reason

Street Drugs

Name	Amount/Day	Reason

Alcohol

Name	Amount/Day/Week	Reason

Substance History and Assessment Tool

1. When you were growing up, did anyone in your family use substances (alcohol or drugs)? If yes, how did the substance use affect the family?

2. When (how old) did you use your first substance (e.g., alcohol, cannabis) and what was it?

3. How long have you been using a substance(s) regularly? Weeks, months, years?

4. Pattern of abuse
   a. When do you use substances?
   b. How much and how often do you use?
   c. Where are you when you use substances and with whom?

5. When did you last use; what was it and how much did you use?

6. Has substance use caused you any problems with family, friends, job, school, the legal system, other? If yes, describe:

7. Have you ever had an injury or accident because of substance abuse? If yes, describe:

8. Have you ever been arrested for a DUI because of your drinking or other substance use?

9. Have you ever been arrested or placed in jail because of drugs or alcohol?

10. Have you ever experienced memory loss the morning after substance use (can't remember what you did the night before)? Describe the event and feelings about the situation:

11. Have you ever tried to stop your substance use? If yes, why were you not able to stop? Did you have any physical symptoms such as shakiness, sweating, nausea, headaches, insomnia, or seizures?

12. Describe a typical day in your life.

13. Are there any changes you would like to make in your life? If so, describe:

14. What plans or ideas do you have for making these changes?

15. History of withdrawal:
    Other comments:

Modified from Townsend 5th ed., 2010, with permission

Short Michigan Alcohol Screening Test (SMAST)

- Do you feel you are a normal drinker? [no] Y__ N__
- Does someone close to you worry about your drinking? [yes] Y__ N__
- Do you feel guilty about your drinking? [yes] Y__ N__
- Do friends/relatives think you're a normal drinker? [no] Y__ N__
- Can you stop drinking when you want to? [no] Y__ N__
- Have you ever attended an AA meeting? [yes] Y__ N__
- Has drinking created problems between you and a loved one/relative? [yes] Y__ N__
- Gotten in trouble at work because of drinking? [yes] Y__ N__
- Neglected obligations/family/work 2 days in a row because of drinking? [yes] Y__ N__
- Gone to anyone for help for your drinking? [yes] Y__ N__
- Ever been in a hospital because of drinking? [yes] Y__ N__
- Arrested for drunk driving or DUI? [yes] Y__ N__
- Arrested for other drunken behavior? [yes] Y__ N__
- Total =

Five or more positive items suggest alcohol problem.
(Positive answers are in brackets above) (Selzer 1975)

(Reprinted with permission from Journal of Studies on Alcohol, vol. 36, pp. 117–126, 1975. Copyright by Journal of Studies on Alcohol, Inc., Rutgers Center of Alcohol Studies, Piscataway, NJ 08854 and Melvin L. Selzer, MD)

DSM-5 Projected elimination of law enforcement encounters from the DSM-5 because of negative association and lack of legal uniformity state to state and among counties.

Mental Status Assessment and Tool

The components of the mental status assessment are:

- General Appearance
- Behavior/Activity
- Speech and Language
- Mood and Affect
- Thought Process and Content
- Perceptual Disturbances
- Memory/Cognitive
- Judgment and Insight

Each component must be approached in a methodical manner so that a thorough evaluation of the client can be done from a mood, thought, appearance, insight, judgment, and overall perspective. It is important to document all these findings even though this record represents one point in time. It is helpful over time to see any patterns (regressions/improvement) and to gain an understanding of any changes that would trigger a need to reevaluate the client or suggest a decline in functioning.

Mental Status Assessment Tool

Identifying Information

Name	Age
Sex	Race/Ethnicity
Significant Other	Educational Level
Religion	Occupation

Presenting problem:

Appearance

Grooming/dress ____________________

Hygiene ____________________

Eye contact ____________________

Continued

Mental Status Assessment Tool—cont'd

Posture ______________________________

Identifying features (marks/scars/tattoos) ______________________________

Appearance versus stated age ______________________________

Overall appearance ______________________________

CLINICAL PEARL: It is helpful to ask the client to talk about him/herself and to *ask open-ended questions* to help the client express thoughts and feelings; e.g., "Tell me why you are here?" Encourage further discussion with: "Tell me more." A less direct and more conversational tone at the beginning of the interview may help reduce the client's anxiety and set the stage for the trust needed in a therapeutic relationship.

Behavior/Activity (check if present)

Hyperactive ______________________________

Agitated ______________________________

Psychomotor retardation ______________________________

Calm ______________________________

Tremors ______________________________

Tics ______________________________

Unusual movements/gestures ______________________________

Catatonia ______________________________

Akathisia ______________________________

Rigidity ______________________________

Facial movements (jaw/lip smacking) ______________________________

Other ______________________________

Speech

Slow/rapid ______________________________

Pressured ______________________________

Tone ______________________________

Volume (loud/soft) ______________________________

Fluency (mute/hesitation/latency of response) ______________________________

Continued

Attitude

Is client:

Cooperative ________ Uncooperative ________

Warm/friendly ________ Distant ________

Suspicious ________ Combative ________

Guarded ________ Aggressive ________

Hostile ________ Aloof ________

Apathetic ________ Other ________

Mood and Affect

Is client:

Elated ________ Sad ________ Depressed ________

Irritable ________ Anxious ________

Fearful ________ Guilty ________

Worried ________ Angry ________

Hopeless ________ Labile ________

Mixed (anxious and depressed) ________

Is client's affect:

Flat ________

Blunted or diminished ________

Appropriate ________

Inappropriate/incongruent (sad and smiling/laughing) ________

____

Other ________

Thought Process

Concrete thinking ________

Circumstantiality ________

Tangentiality ________

Loose association ________

Echolalia ________

Flight of ideas ________

Perseveration ________

Clang associations ________

Blocking ________

Continued

Word salad ______________________________

Derailment ______________________________

Other ______________________________

Thought Content

Does client have:

Delusions (grandiose/persecution/reference/somatic): ______________

____

Suicidal/homicidal thoughts ______________________________

If homicidal, toward whom? (Must report and notify intended victim)

____

Obsessions______________________________

Paranoia ______________________________

Phobias ______________________________

Magical thinking ______________________________

Poverty of speech ______________________________

Other ______________________________

CLINICAL PEARL: Questions around suicide and homicide need to be direct. For instance, *Are you thinking of harming yourself/another person right now?* (If another, who?) Clients will usually admit to suicidal thoughts *if asked directly* but will not always volunteer this information. Any threat to harm someone else requires informing the potential victim and the authorities. *(See When Confidentiality Must be Breached, Tarasoff Principle/Duty to Warn, in Basics Tab.)*

Perceptual Disturbances

Is client experiencing:

Visual Hallucinations ______________________________

Auditory Hallucinations ______________________________

Commenting ______________________________

Discussing ______________________________

Commanding ______________________________

Loud ______________________________

Soft ______________________________

Other ______________________________

Other Hallucination (olfactory/tactile) ______________________________

Continued

Illusions ______________________

Depersonalization ______________________

Other ______________________

Memory/Cognitive

Orientation (time/place/person)______________________

Memory (recent/remote/confabulation) ______________________

Level of alertness ______________________

Insight and Judgment

Insight (awareness of the nature of the illness)______________________

Judgment ______________________

For example: "What would you do if you saw a fire in a movie theater?"

Other ______________________

Impulse control ______________________

Other ______________________

DSM-IV-TR Multiaxial Classification and Tool

Allows for assessment on various axes, which provides information on different domains and assists in planning interventions and identifying outcomes. Includes GAF (axis V) (explained later).

Components

Axis I: Clinical Disorder (or focus of clinical attention)
Axis II: Personality Disorders/Mental Retardation
Axis III: General Medical Conditions
Axis IV: Psychosocial/Environmental
Axis V: Global Assessment of Functioning (GAF)
Current:
Past Year, highest level:
Admission:
Discharge:

Sample DSM-IV-TR Multiaxial Classifications

Axis I: V61.10 Partner Relational Problem
Axis II: 301.6 Dependent Personality Disorder
Axis III: 564.1 Irritable Bowel Syndrome
Axis IV: Two small daughters at home
Axis V: GAF (current) 65
Past year, highest level: 80

Axis I: 296.44 Bipolar I Disorder, most recent episode manic, severe with psychotic features
Axis II: 301.83 Borderline Personality Disorder
Axis III: 704.00 Alopecia
Axis IV: Unemployed
Axis V: GAF Admission: 28
Discharge: 62

DSM-IV-TR Multiaxial Evaluation Tool*

Axis I:
Clinical Disorder/Clinical Focus
Include diagnostic code/
DSM-IV name

Axis II:
Personality Disorders/Mental Retardation; include
Diagnostic code/DSM-IV name

Axis III:
Any General Medical Conditions
Include ICD-9-CM codes/names

Axis IV:
Psychosocial/Environmental Problems:
(family/primary support group/social/occupational/ educational/health care/legal/crime/other)

Axis V (GAF):
Current/hospital:
Highest level past year/discharge:

*See *Tools Tab* for DSM-IV-TR Classification/Codes

CLINICAL PEARL: It is often an Axis I disorder (depression/anxiety) that brings a client into therapy but an Axis II disorder (dependent/borderline personality) that keeps the client in therapy. Problems/crises continue in spite of treatment.

Global Assessment of Functioning (GAF)/Scale

The GAF provides an *overall* rating of assessment of function. It is concerned with psychosocial/occupational aspects and divided into ten ranges of functioning, covering both *symptom severity* and *functioning*. The GAF is recorded as a numerical value on Axis V of the Multiaxial System (see above).

Global Assessment of Functioning (GAF) Scale

Code	**Note: Use intermediate codes when appropriate (e.g., 45, 68, 72)**
100 91	Superior functioning in a wide range of activities, life's problems never seem to get out of hand, sought out by others because of his or her many positive qualities. No symptoms.
90 81	Absent or minimal symptoms (e.g., mild anxiety before an exam), good functioning in all areas, interested and involved in a wide range of activities, socially effective; generally satisfied with life; no more than general problems or concerns (e.g., an occasional argument with family members).
80 71	If symptoms are present, they are transient and expectable reactions to psychosocial stressors (e.g., difficulty concentrating after family argument); slight impairment in social, work, or school functioning (e.g., temporarily falling behind in schoolwork).
70 61	Some mild symptoms (e.g., depressed mood and mild insomnia) OR some difficulty in social, occupational, or school functioning (e.g., occasional truancy, or theft within the household), but generally functioning pretty well, has some meaningful interpersonal relationships.
60 51	Moderate symptoms (e.g., flat affect and circumstantial speech, occasional panic attacks) OR moderate difficulty in social, occupational, or school functioning (e.g., few friends, conflicts with peers or co-workers).
50 41	Serious symptoms (e.g., suicidal ideation, severe obsessional rituals, frequent shoplifting) OR serious impairment in social, occupational, or school functioning (e.g., no friends, unable to keep a job).

Continued

Global Assessment of Functioning (GAF) Scale—cont'd

Code	**Note: Use intermediate codes when appropriate (e.g., 45, 68, 72)**
40 31	Some impairment in reality testing or communication (e.g., speech is at times illogical, obscure, or irrelevant) OR major impairment in several areas, such as work, school, family relations, judgment, thinking, or mood (e.g., depressed man avoids friends, neglects family, and is unable to work; child frequently beats up younger children, is defiant at home, and is failing at school).
30 21	Behavior is considerably influenced by delusions or hallucinations OR serious impairment in communication or judgment (e.g., sometimes incoherent, acts grossly inappropriately, suicidal preoccupation) OR inability to function in almost all areas (e.g., stays in bed all day; no job, home, or friends).
20 11	Some danger of hurting self or others (e.g., suicide attempts without clear expectation of death; frequently violent; manic excitement) OR occasionally fails to maintain minimal personal hygiene (e.g., smears feces) OR gross impairment in communication (e.g., largely incoherent or mute).
10 1	Persistent danger of severely hurting self or others (e.g., recurrent violence) OR persistent inability to maintain minimal personal hygiene OR serious suicidal act with clear expectation of death.

0 = Inadequate information

Abnormal Involuntary Movement Scale (AIMS)

- AIMS is a 5- to 10-minute clinician/other-trained rater (psychiatric nurse) scale to assess for tardive dyskinesia. AIMS is not a scored scale but rather a comparative scale documenting changes over time (Guy 1976).
- Baseline should be done before instituting pharmacotherapy and then every 3 to 6 months thereafter. Check with federal and hospital regulations for time frames. Long-term care facilities are required to perform the AIMS at initiation of antipsychotic therapy and every 6 months thereafter.

AIMS Examination Procedure

Either before or after completing the examination procedure, observe the client unobtrusively, at rest (e.g., in waiting room). The chair to be used in this examination should be hard and firm without arms.

- Ask client to remove shoes and socks.
- Ask client if there is anything in his/her mouth (e.g., gum, candy); if there is, to remove it.
- Ask client about the current condition of his/her teeth. Ask client if he/she wears dentures. Do teeth or dentures bother the client now?
- Ask client whether he/she notices any movements in mouth, face, hands, or feet. If yes, ask to describe and to what extent they currently bother client or interfere with his/her activities.
- Have client sit in chair with hands on knees, legs slightly apart and feet flat on floor. (Look at entire body for movements while client is in this position.)
- Ask client to sit with hands hanging unsupported: if male, between legs; if female and wearing a dress, hanging over knees. (Observe hands and other body areas.)
- Ask client to open mouth. (Observe tongue at rest in mouth.) Do this twice.
- Ask client to protrude tongue. (Observe abnormalities of tongue movement.) Do this twice.
- Ask client to tap thumb, with each finger, as rapidly as possible for 10 to 15 seconds; separately with right hand, then with left hand. (Observe facial and leg movements.)
- Flex and extend client's left and right arms (one at a time). (Note any rigidity.)
- Ask client to stand up. (Observe in profile. Observe all body areas again, hips included.)
- Ask client to extend both arms outstretched in front with palms down. (Observe trunk, legs, and mouth.)
- Have client walk a few paces, turn, and walk back to chair. (Observe hands and gait.) Do this twice.

AIMS Rating Form	
Name	Rater Name
Date	ID #
Instructions: Complete the above examination procedure before making ratings. For movement ratings, circle the highest severity observed.	Code: 0: None 1: Minimal, may be extreme normal 2: Mild 3: Moderate 4: Severe

Continued

AIMS Rating Form—cont'd

Facial and Oral Movements	**1. Muscles of Facial Expression** • e.g., movements of forehead, eyebrows, periorbital area, cheeks • include frowning, blinking, smiling, and grimacing	0 1 2 3 4
	2. Lips and Perioral Area • e.g., puckering, pouting, smacking	0 1 2 3 4
	3. Jaw • e.g., biting, clenching, chewing, mouth opening, lateral movement	0 1 2 3 4
	4. Tongue • Rate only increase in movements both in and out of the mouth, NOT the inability to sustain movement	0 1 2 3 4
Extremity Movements	**5. Upper** *(arms, wrists, hands, fingers)* • Include choreic movements (i.e., rapid, objectively purposeless, irregular, spontaneous), athetoid movements (i.e., slow, irregular, complex, serpentine). • Do NOT include tremor (i.e., repetitive, regular, rhythmic).	0 1 2 3 4
Trunk Movements	**6. Lower** *(legs, knees, ankles, toes)* • e.g., lateral knee movement, foot tapping, heel dropping, foot squirming, inversion and eversion of the foot	0 1 2 3 4
	7. Neck, shoulders, hips • e.g., rocking, twisting, squirming, pelvic gyrations	0 1 2 3 4
Global Judgments	**8. Severity of Abnormal Movements**	0 1 2 3 4
	9. Incapacitation Due to Abnormal Movements	0 1 2 3 4
	10. Client's Awareness of Abnormal Movements • Rate only client's report.	0 1 2 3 4

Continued

AIMS Rating Form—cont'd

Dental Status	**11. Current Problems With Teeth and/or Dentures**	0: No 1: Yes
	12. Does Client Usually Wear Dentures?	0: No 1: Yes

The Edinburgh Postnatal Depression Scale (EPDS)

The EPDS is a valid screening tool for detecting postpartum depression. It is important to differentiate postpartum blues from postpartal depression and to observe for psychosis. Bipolar disorder and previous postpartum psychosis increase risk for suicide or infanticide. (See *Postpartum Major Depressive Episode* in the Disorders-Interventions Tab for signs and symptoms, evaluation, and treatment of postpartum depression.) **Note:** May also be used to screen for paternal depression (Edmondson 2010).

The Edinburgh Postnatal Depression Scale (EPDS)

Name: ______________________

Your date of birth: ______________________

Baby's Age: ______________________

As you have recently had a baby, we would like to know how you are feeling now. Please underline the answer that comes closest to how you have felt IN THE PAST 7 DAYS, not just how you feel today.

Sample question:

Here is an example already completed:

I have felt happy

- Yes, most of the time
- Yes, some of the time
- No, not very often
- No, not at all

This would mean "I have felt happy some of the time during the past week."

Please complete the following questions in the same way:

1. I have been able to laugh and see the funny side of things
   - As much as I always could
   - Not quite so much now
   - Definitely not so much now
   - Not at all
2. I have looked forward with enjoyment to things.
   - As much as I ever did
   - Rather less than I used to
   - Definitely less than I used to
   - Hardly at all

Continued

The Edinburgh Postnatal Depression Scale (EPDS)—cont'd

3. I have blamed myself unnecessarily when things went wrong.*
   - Yes, most of the time
   - Yes, some of the time
   - Not very often
   - No, never

4. I have been anxious or worried for no good reason.
   - No, not at all
   - Hardly ever
   - Yes, sometimes
   - Yes, very often

5. I have felt scared or panicky for no very good reason.*
   - Yes, quite a lot
   - Yes, sometimes
   - No, not much
   - No, not at all

6. Things have been getting on top of me.*
   - Yes, most of the time I haven't been able to cope at all
   - Yes, sometimes I haven't been coping as well as usual
   - No, most of the time I have coped quite well
   - No, I have been coping as well as ever

7. I have been so unhappy that I have had difficulty sleeping.*
   - Yes, most of the time
   - Yes, sometimes
   - Not very often
   - No, not at all

8. I have felt sad or miserable.*
   - Yes, most of the time
   - Yes, quite often
   - Not very often
   - No, not at all

9. I have been so unhappy that I have been crying.*
   - Yes, most of the time
   - Yes, quite often
   - Only occasionally
   - No, never

10. The thought of harming myself has occurred to me.*
    - Yes, quite often
    - Sometimes
    - Hardly ever
    - Never

Total score = ______ (See scoring on following page)

Instructions for users:

1. The mother is asked to underline the response that comes closest to how she has been feeling in the previous 7 days.

2. All ten items must be completed.

3. Care should be taken to avoid the possibility of the mother discussing her answers with others.

4. The mother should complete the scale herself, unless she has limited English or has difficulty with reading.

5. The EPDS may be used at 6–8 weeks to screen postnatal women. The child health clinic, postnatal check-up, or a home visit may provide suitable opportunities for its completion.

Scoring:

Questions 1, 2, and 4 are scored 0, 1, 2, and 3 according to increased severity of the symptoms. The top response (e.g., As much as I always could, question 1) would be scored a 0 and the bottom response (e.g., Not at all, question 1) scored a 3. Items marked with an asterisk * (questions 3, 5–10) are reverse scored (i.e., 3, 2, 1, and 0). The total score is calculated by adding together the scores for each of the ten items. Maximum score is 30. Patients scoring 13 or more should be assessed for possible depression. A cut-off of 10 or more may be used if greater sensitivity is required. Any score above 0 on item 10 should always prompt further assessment.

Translations of the scale, and guidance as to its use, may be found in Cox JL, Holden J. Perinatal Mental Health: A Guide to the Edinburgh Postnatal Depression Scale. London: Gaskell, 2003.

Scoring for Men:

A score of greater than 10 was found to be the optimal cutoff for men and shown to have a reasonable sensitivity and specificity (Edmondson 2010).

Depression-Arkansas Scale (D-ARK Scale)

The D-ARK scale is a practical, self-report assessment scale for measuring major depressive disorder in clinical settings. It is scientifically sound and simple to use (Smith, Kramer, Hollenberg et al 2002).

Depression-Arkansas (D-ARK) Scale

Underline or circle your response to each of 11 questions that follow; note that each question relates to the **past 4 weeks**:

1. How often *in the past 4 weeks* have you felt depressed, blue, or in low spirits for most of the day?
   (1) Not at all (2) 1 to 3 days a week (3) Most days a week (4) Nearly every day for at least two weeks

Continued

Depression-Arkansas (D-ARK) Scale—cont'd

2. How often *in the past 4 weeks* did you have days in which you experienced little or no pleasure in most of your activities?
   (1) Not at all (2) 1 to 3 days a week (3) Most days a week (4) Nearly every day for at least two weeks
3. How often *in the past 4 weeks* has your appetite been either less than usual or greater than usual?
   (1) Not at all (2) 1 to 3 days a week (3) Most days a week (4) Nearly every day for at least two weeks
4. *In the past 4 weeks,* have you gained or lost weight without trying to?
   (1) No (2) Yes, a little weight (3) Yes, some weight (4) Yes, a lot of weight
5. How often *in the past 4 weeks* have you had difficulty sleeping or trouble with sleeping too much?
   (1) Not at all (2) 1 to 3 days a week (3) Most days a week (4) Nearly every day for at least two weeks
6. *In the past 4 weeks,* has your physical activity been slowed down or speeded up so much people who know you could notice?
   (1) No (2) Yes, a little slowed or speeded up (3) Yes, somewhat slowed or speeded up (4) Yes, very slowed or speeded up
7. *In the past 4 weeks,* have you often felt more tired out or less energetic than usual?
   (1) No (2) Yes, a little tired (3) Yes, somewhat tired out (4) Yes, very tired out
8. How often *in the past 4 weeks* have you felt worthless or been bothered by feelings of guilt?
   (1) Not at all (2) 1 to 3 days a week (3) Most days a week (4) Nearly every day for at least two weeks
9. *In the past 4 weeks,* have you often had trouble thinking, concentrating, or making decisions?
   (1) No (2) Yes, a little trouble thinking (3) Yes, some trouble thinking (4) Yes, a lot of trouble thinking
10. How often have you thought about death or suicide *in the past 4 weeks?*
    (1) Not at all (2) 1 to 3 days a week (3) Most days a week (4) Nearly every day for at least two weeks
11. *In the past 4 weeks,* have you thought a lot about a specific way to commit suicide?
    (1) No (2) Yes

Continued

Depression-Arkansas (D-ARK) Scale—cont'd

Diagnostic Score (see scoring below)
Part A ____________
Part B ____________
Total Score (A + B) = ____________

D-ARK Diagnostic Scoring

Part A: If respondent scores Questions 1 or 2 *greater than or equal to 2;* then Part A = 1

Part B: Score individual items as follows:

If question 1 is greater than or equal to 2, *Criterion 1* = 1;
Score ____________

If question 2 is greater than or equal to 2, *Criterion 2* = 1;
Score ____________

If question 3 is greater than or equal to 2, *or* Question 4 is greater than or equal to 2, *Criterion 3* = 1;
Score ____________

If questions 5–9 are greater than or equal to 3, *Criteria 4–8* = 1 each;
Score ____________

If Question 10 is greater than or equal to 3, *or* Question 11 = 2, *Criterion 9* = 1;
Score ____________

Part B: Add scores for Criterion 1 through 9, and Total: ______; if the total of Criteria 1–9 is *greater than or equal to 5,* then Part B = 1

If Part A = 1 and Part B = 1, then the respondent meets the criteria for depression.

Note: The D-ARK Scale includes all 9 DSM-IV Criteria symptoms for diagnosing Major Depressive Disorder. *(See DSM-IV-TR, Mood Episodes, Criteria for Major Depressive Episode and also Major Depressive Episode in the Disorders-Interventions Tab.)*

D-ARK Severity Scoring

Recode Questions 1–10 as 0 to 3; if Question 11 = 1, then Question 11 = 0; if Question 11 = 2, then Question 11 = 3. Calculate the mean of questions 1–11; multiply by 33.33. This product is the severity score. If Question 10 is missing (not answered) or two or more questions are missing, do not score severity.

Geriatric Depression Rating Scale (GDS)

Short Version

Choose the best answer for how you have felt over the past week (circle yes or no):

1. Are you basically satisfied with your life? YES/**NO**
2. Have you dropped many of your activities and interests? **YES**/NO
3. Do you feel that your life is empty? **YES**/NO
4. Do you often get bored? **YES**/NO
5. Are you in good spirits most of the time? YES/**NO**
6. Are you afraid that something bad is going to happen to you? **YES**/NO
7. Do you feel happy most of the time? YES/**NO**
8. Do you often feel helpless? **YES**/NO
9. Do you prefer to stay at home, rather than going out and doing new things? **YES**/NO
10. Do you feel you have more problems with memory than most? **YES**/NO
11. Do you think it is wonderful to be alive now? YES/**NO**
12. Do you feel pretty worthless the way you are now? **YES**/NO
13. Do you feel full of energy? YES/**NO**
14. Do you feel that your situation is hopeless? **YES**/NO
15. Do you think that most people are better off than you are? **YES**/NO

Total Score =

Bold answers = depression

GDS Scoring:

12–15 Severe depression

8–11 Moderate depression

5–7 Mild depression

0–4 Normal

(Yesavage et al 1983; Sheikh 1986; GDS Web site: http://www.stanford.edu/~yesavage/)

ALERT: As with all rating scales, further evaluation and monitoring are often needed. Be sure to perform a Mini-Mental State Examination (MMSE) first to screen for/rule out dementia (cognitive deficits).

Mood Disorder Questionnaire

The Mood Disorder Questionnaire (MDQ) is a useful screening tool for bipolar spectrum disorder in an outpatient population. A score of 7 or more yielded a good sensitivity (0.73) and a very good specificity (0.90).

1. Has there ever been a period of time when you were not your usual self (while not using drugs or alcohol) and ...		
...you felt so good or so hyper that other people thought you were not your normal self, or you were so hyper that you got into trouble? (circle yes or no for each line, please)	Yes	No
...you were so irritable that you shouted at people or started arguments?	Yes	No
...you felt much more self-confident than usual?	Yes	No
...you got much less sleep than usual and found you didn't really miss it?	Yes	No
...you were much more talkative or spoke faster than usual?	Yes	No
...thoughts raced through your head or you couldn't slow your mind down?	Yes	No
...you were so easily distracted by things around you that you had trouble concentrating or staying on track?	Yes	No
...you had much more energy than usual?	Yes	No
...you were much more active or did many more things than usual?	Yes	No
...you were much more social or outgoing than usual; for example, you telephoned friends in the middle of the night?	Yes	No
...you were much more interested in sex than usual?	Yes	No
...you did things that were unusual for you or that other people might have thought were excessive, foolish, or risky?	Yes	No
...spending money got you or your family into trouble?	Yes	No
Total number of "Yes" responses to question 1	________	
2. If you checked YES to more than one of the above, have several of these ever happened during the **same period of time?**	Yes	No
3. How much of a **problem** did any of these cause you – like being unable to work; having family, money, or legal troubles; getting into arguments or fights?	No problem Minor problem Moderate problem Serious problem	

Scoring:
An individual is considered positive for Bipolar Disorder if they answered:

1. "Yes" to at least 7 of the 13 items in question 1 AND
2. "Yes" to question number 2 AND
3. "Moderate" or "Serious" to question number 3.

All three of the criteria should be met. A positive screen indicates that the person should receive a comprehensive diagnostic evaluation for bipolar spectrum disorder by a psychiatrist, licensed psychologist, or advanced practice psychiatric nurse.

From Hirschfeld R, Williams JB, Spitzer RL et al. Development and validation of a screening instrument for bipolar spectrum disorder: The Mood Disorder Questionnaire. Am J Psychiatry 2000; 157:1873–1875. Reprinted with permission from Dr. Robert MA Hirschfeld.

Mini-Mental State Examination (MMSE)

The *Mini-Mental State Examination* is a brief (10-minute) standardized, reliable screening instrument used to assess for cognitive impairment and commonly used to screen for dementia. It evaluates orientation, registration, concentration, language, short-term memory, and visual-spatial aspects and can be scored quickly (24–30 = normal; 18–23 = mild/moderate cognitive impairment; 0–17 = severe cognitive impairment). (Folstein et al 1975; Psychological Assessment Resources, Inc.)

The Clock-Drawing Test

Another test that is said to be possibly more sensitive to *early* dementia is the clock-drawing test. There are many variations and clock is first drawn (by clinician) and divided into tenths or quadrants. Client is asked to put the numbers in the appropriate places and then indicate the time as "ten minutes after eleven." Scoring is based on test used and completion of the tasks (Manos 2004).

Ethnocultural Considerations

With over 400 ethnocultural groups, it is impossible to cover every group within North America. It is important, however, to become familiar with the characteristics and customs of most ethnocultural groups you will be working with and sensitive to any differences.

Ethnicity refers to a common ancestry through which individuals have evolved shared values and customs. This sense of commonality is transmitted over generations by family and reinforced by the surrounding community (McGoldrick, 2005).

Suggested References for Further Reading Include:

McGoldrick M, Giordano J, Garcia-Preto N. Ethnicity and Family Therapy, 3rd ed. New York: The Guilford Press, 2005

Purnell LD, Paulanka BJ. Guide to Culturally Competent Health Care, 2nd ed. Philadelphia: FA Davis, 2009

Purnell LD, Paulanka BJ. Transcultural Health Care: A Culturally Competent Approach, 3rd ed. Philadelphia: FA Davis, 2008

Culturally Mediated Beliefs and Practices

	Dying/birth	Role Differences	Religion	Communication
African American	Reluctant to donate organs Ask about advance directives/durable power of attorney (may not have any) – usually family makes decisions as a whole. Burials may take up to 5–7 d after death. Varied responses to death.	Varies by educational level/socioeconomic level. High percentage of families is matriarchal. Extended family important in health education; include women in decision making/health information.	Baptist/Methodist/other Protestant/Muslim (Nation of Islam/other sects) Determine affiliation during interview/determine importance of church/religion.	*Eye Contact:* Demonstrates respect/trust, but direct contact may be interpreted as aggressive. *Other:* Silence may indicate distrust. Prefer use of last name (upon greeting) unless referred to otherwise.
Arab American	Colostrum is believed harmful to the infant Death is God's will; turn patient's bed to face Mecca and read the Koran. No cremation, no autopsy (except forensic) and organ donation acceptable.	Men make most decisions (patrilineal) and women responsible for daily needs (wield a lot of influence over family and home); family loyalty more important than individual needs.	Muslim (usually Sunni)/Protestant/Greek orthodox/other Christian. Duties of Islam: Declaration of faith, prayer 5 times/d, alms-giving, fasting during Ramadan, and pilgrimage to Mecca.	*Eye Contact:* Females may avoid eye contact with males/strangers. *Other:* Supportive family members may need a break from caregiving; obtain an interpreter if necessary.

Continued

Culturally Mediated Beliefs and Practices—cont'd

	Dying/birth	Role Differences	Religion	Communication
Asian American	May use incense/ spiritual. Need extra time with deceased members; natural cycle of life.	Father/eldest son primary decision maker; recognized head has great authority.	Primarily Buddhism and Catholicism; Taoism and Islam	*Eye Contact:* Direct eye contact may be viewed as disrespectful. *Other:* Use interpreters whenever possible (be careful about tone of voice). Often a formal distance.
Native Americans	Full family involvement throughout life cycle; do not practice birth control or limit size of family.	Varies tribe to tribe; most tribes matrilineal and be sure to identify the gate-keeper of the tribe.	Traditional Native American or Christian; spirituality based on harmony with nature.	*Eye Contact:* Eye contact sustained. *Other:* American Indian may be term preferred by older adults; use an interpreter to avoid misunderstandings. Do not point with finger.

Continued

Culturally Mediated Beliefs and Practices—cont'd

	Dying/birth	Role Differences	Religion	Communication
Mexican Americans	Family support during labor; very expressive during bereavement (find a place where family can grieve together quietly). Fertility practices follow Catholic teachings. Abortion considered wrong.	Equal decision making with all family members; men expected to provide financial support.	Roman Catholic primarily	*Eye Contact:* Eye contact may be avoided with authority figures. *Other:* Silence may indicate disagreement with proposed plan of care; greet adults formally (señor, señora, etc, unless told otherwise).
Russian Americans	Father may not attend birth; usually closest family female does; family wants to be informed of impending death before patient.	Men and women share decision making; family, women, children highly valued.	Eastern Orthodox and Judaism; remember recent oppression; also Molokans, Tartar Muslims, Pentecostals, Baptists. About 60% not religious	*Eye Contact*: Direct eye contact acceptable/nodding means approval. *Other:* Use interpreters whenever possible; Russians are distant until trust is established.

Adapted from Purnell & Paulanka 2008 and Myers 2010, with permission

Perception of Mental Health Services: Ethnocultural Differences

African Americans

- Often distrustful of therapy and mental health services. May seek therapy because of child-focused concerns.
- Seek help and support through "the church," which provides a sense of belonging and community (social activities/choir). Therapy is for "crazy people" (McGoldrick 2005).

Mexican Americans

- Understanding the migration of the family is important, including who has been left behind. The church in the barrio often provides community support.
- Curanderos (folk healers) may be consulted for problems such as: mal de ojo (evil eye) and susto (fright) (McGoldrick 2005).

Puerto Ricans

- Nominally Catholic, most value the spirit and soul. Many believe in spirits that protect or harm and the value of incense and candles to ward off the "evil eye."
- Often underutilize mental health services, and therapist needs to understand that expectations about outcome may differ (McGoldrick 2005).

Asian American

- Many Asian-American families are transitioning from the extended family to the nuclear unit and struggling to hold on to old ways while developing new skills.
- Six predictors of mental health problems are: 1) employment/financial status, 2) gender (women more vulnerable), 3) old age, 4) social isolation, 5) recent immigration, and 6) refugee premigration experiences and post-migration adjustment (McGoldrick 2005).

Above are just a few examples of many ethnocultural groups and the differences in the understanding and perception of mental health/therapy. Please refer to suggested references (p. 50) for additional and more comprehensive information.

Ethnocultural Assessment Tool

Client's name	Ethnic origin
City/State	Birth date
Significant other	Relationship
Primary language spoken	Second language
Interpreter required?	Available?
Highest level of education	Occupation
Presenting problem/chief complaint:	

Has problem occurred before? If so how was it handled?
Client's usual manner of coping with stress?
Who is (are) client's main support system?
Family living arrangements (describe):
Major decision maker in family:
Client's/family members' roles in the family:
Religious beliefs and practices:
Are there religious restrictions or requirements?
Who takes responsibility for health concerns in family?
Any special health concerns or beliefs?
Who does family usually approach for medical assistance?
Usual emotional/behavioral response to:

Anger____

Anxiety____

Pain____

Fear____

Loss/change/failure__________________________________

Sensitive topics client unwilling to discuss due to ethnocultural taboos?
Client's feelings about touch and touching?
Client's feelings regarding eye contact?
Client's orientation to time (past/present/future)?
Illnesses/diseases common to client's ethnicity?
Client's favorite foods:

Foods that client requests or refuses because of ethnocultural reasons:
Client's perception of the problem and expectations of care and outcome:
Other:

Modified from Townsend 5th ed., 2010, with permission

Documentation

Problem-Oriented Record (POR)

POR	Data	Nursing Process
S (Subjective)	Client's verbal reports (e.g., "I feel nervous")	Assessment
O (Objective)	Observation (e.g., client is pacing)	Assessment
A (Assessment)	Evaluation/interpretation of S and O	Diagnosis/outcome identification
P (Plan)	Actions to resolve problem	Planning
I (Intervention)	Descriptions of actions completed	Implementation
E (Evaluation)	Reassessment to determine results and necessity of new plan of action	Evaluation

Focus Charting (DAR)

Charting	Data	Nursing Process
D (Data)	Describes observations about client/supports the stated focus	Assessment
Focus	Current client concern/behavior/ significant change in client status	Diagnosis/outcome identification
A (Action)	Immediate/future actions	Plan and implementation
R (Response)	Client's response to care or therapy	Evaluation

PIE Method (APIE)

Charting	Data	Nursing Process
A (Assessment)	Subjective and objective data collected at each shift	Assessment
P (Problem)	Problems being addressed from written problem list and identified outcomes	Diagnosis/outcome identification
I (intervention)	Actions performed directed at problem resolution	Plan and implementation
E (Evaluation)	Response appraisal to determine intervention effectiveness	Evaluation

POR, DAR, and APIE modified from Townsend 5th ed., 2010, with permission

CLINICAL PEARL: It is important to systematically assess and evaluate all clients and to develop a plan of action, reevaluating all outcomes. It is equally important to document all assessments, plans, treatments, and outcomes. You may "know" you provided competent treatment, but without documentation there is *no record* from a legal perspective. *Do not ever become complacent about documentation.*

Example of APIE Charting

DATE/TIME	PROBLEM	PROGRESS NOTE
5–22–11 1000	Social Isolation	*A:* States he does not want to sit with or talk to others; they "frighten him." Stays in room; no social involvement. *P:* Social isolation due to inability to trust. *I:* Spent time alone with client to initiate trust; accompanied client to group activities; praised participation. *E:* Cooperative although still uncomfortable in presence of group; accepted positive feedback.

Example modified from Townsend 5th ed., 2010, with permission

Psychiatric Disorders/Interventions

Psychiatric Disorders

Psychiatric Interventions

DSM-5: Preview of Changes to Come

The DSM-5, which has been years in the making, will reflect a major overhaul of the current revision, the DSM-IV-TR (2000). Note the change from DSM-V (Roman numeral) to DSM-5. The first DSM I published (1952) with revisions in between through 2000. However, research and knowledge in the areas of neuroscience, genetics, and behavior have significantly expanded in the past decade to require a thorough review and restructuring in DSM-5, with a continued focus on clinical utility as well as evidence-based practice. DSM-5 is projected to publish in May of 2013. Some of the notable changes include how clients will be assessed and it will focus on *measurement-based care* (dsm5.org 2011; DSM-V 2009).

- The DSM-5 is considering the use of **"dimensional assessments,"** which will consider all the symptoms the client is presenting, rather than **categorizing** a client based solely on meeting one set of criteria for a "specific disorder." This would allow clinicians (including primary care clinicians) to identify the presence of symptoms and **rate** their **severity**. One would then be able to track progress against this baseline.
- **Cross-cutting assessments** would allow clinicians to measure symptoms (not necessarily a part of any diagnostic criteria) that *cross over many disorders* (depressed mood, anxiety, substance use, anger). The focus is on brief and simple rating scales (4–5 point scales) for use in all clinical settings, such as *suicide risk scales* to identify early on those at risk, using research-based criteria.
- **Assessment levels** – There may be different levels of assessment. **Level 1** could be simple and denote if symptoms are clinically significant for a Level 2 assessment. Ratings may be by patient, informant, or clinician. Level 2 assessment scales could be clinician-rated scales or scales currently in development at the National Institutes of Health. The NIH has developed several assessments as part of a **Patient-Reported Outcome Measurement Information System (PROMIS)** (www.nihpromis.org).

Some areas under consideration for change within diagnostic categories include (DSM-5.org 2011):

- **Delirium, Dementia, and Amnestic Disorders**
  - Removing the term *Dementia* and adding to the DSM-5: Major Neurocognitive Disorders, Minor Neurocognitive Disorders, and including Dementia of the Alzheimer's type as a subtype of major neurocognitive disorder.
- **Substance-Related Disorders**
  - Discussions are underway to eliminate *substance abuse* and *dependence* to highlight the distinction between "drug-seeking addictive behavior" and normal physiologic tolerance to prescribed drugs (opioids), including withdrawal. The new category may be titled, *addictions and related disorders.*

- *Substance-use disorders* would identify the specific drug (e.g., cocaine-use disorder, alcohol-use disorder). *Drug craving* would be added as a criterion for diagnosing addiction. Encounters with the law dropped because of the negative implications and lack of uniformity in state and county laws.
- *Behavioral addictions* will include gambling, but there may not yet be enough research evidence for Internet, eating, shopping, sex, work, etc. as addictions.

Schizophrenia and Other Psychotic Disorders

- There are discussions and proposals for an "attenuated psychotic symptoms syndrome (psychosis risk syndrome)."
- The following are being considered for deletion:
  - 295.30. Schizophrenia – Paranoid Type
  - 295.10. Schizophrenia – Disorganized Type
  - 295.20. Schizophrenia – Catatonic Type
  - 295.90. Schizophrenia – Undifferentiated Type
  - 295.60. Schizophrenia – Residual Type
  - 297.3. Shared Psychotic Disorder

Mood Disorders

- Depressive Disorder NOS to be changed to Depressive Conditions Not Elsewhere Classified, to allow for depressive symptoms that do not meet criteria for a mood disorder.
- Suggested is an *"anxiety dimension"* across all mood disorders as well as a "*suicide assessment dimension*."
- Mood disorders recommended for deletion or reclassification: Mixed episode.
- Mood disorders to be added: Mixed anxiety depression, premenstrual dysmorphic disorder.
- Possible removal: Bipolar I Disorder – most recent episode mixed.
- Possible new diagnostic category – "temper dysregulation with dysphoria." Help differentiate children from bipolar disorder and oppositional defiant disorder.

Anxiety Disorders

- Anxiety disorder possibly to be reclassified: Obsessive-Compulsive Disorder [Anxiety and Obsessive-Compulsive Spectrum Disorders].
- Removal: Agoraphobia without history of panic disorder.
- Additions: Hoarding disorder (including animals), skin picking disorder, olfactory reference disorder, substance-induced (indicate substance) tic disorder, tic due to a general medical condition.

Somatoform Disorders

- Addition: Complex somatic symptom disorder (may now include somatization disorder, hypochondriasis, etc.)
- Body dysmorphic disorder: Reclassification under "anxiety and obsessive-compulsive spectrum disorders."

- **Sexual and Gender Identity Disorders**
  - Additions: Hypersexual disorder, paraphilic coercive disorder, sexual interest/arousal disorder in women and in men, genito-pelvic pain/penetration disorder, and sexual dysfunction due to a general medical condition.
  - Removal: Sexual aversion disorder.
  - Hypoactive sexual desire disorder, several dyspareunias, vaginismus, and others: Subsumed under other diagnoses.
  - Changing the name *gender identity disorder* to *gender incongruence*.
- **Eating Disorders**
  - Eating disorders possibly renamed: "Eating and feeding disorders," for inclusion of feeding disorders that begin in infancy and early childhood, to be renamed: Avoidant/restrictive food intake disorder.
  - New addition (currently in the appendix): Binge eating disorder.
- **Personality Disorders**
  - Aiming to redefine PD, and use of a *dimensional view* of PDs, rather than rigidly categorize them. Focus on dysfunctional traits, such as antagonism and impulsivity. Narcissistic and histrionic may be subsumed under other personality types. Will include *severity levels, five broad types, personality trait domains, specific trait facets*, and a new definition of personality disorder.
  - There have been discussions of making borderline personality disorder an Axis I diagnosis.
- **Disorders of Childhood and Adolescence**
  - Recommend a new category: Autism spectrum disorders (to incorporate current disorders, such as Asperger's, childhood disintegrative disorder, etc.).
  - Recommends using *intellectual disability* to replace mental retardation.
  - Suggested additions include: Posttraumatic stress disorder in preschool children, temper dysregulation disorder with dysphoria, non-suicidal self injury, and others.
  - Proposed reclassification into other diagnostic categories: Pica, feeding disorder of infancy or early childhood, etc.
  - Attention deficit/hyperactivity disorder: Would change diagnostic criteria from symptoms being present before age 7 to before age 12.
- **Multiaxial System** There are discussions around examining the value of Axis III (medical conditions) and the possible collapsing of Axes I, II, and III into one axis covering all psychiatric and medical diagnoses. Axis IV group is examining the ICD 10 codes for possible use. Axis IV is also under review.

Because the DSM-5 remains a "work in progress" the above is meant to present some of the general ideas and discussions taking place within the DSM-5 task force, though they are not yet final and may change. Clearly, the changes are fairly extensive and will require a reintroduction to the new concepts, categories, and diagnoses when DSM-5 publishes. There is also much controversy over the DSM-5 and articles enumerating these concerns have been posted on the Internet (Frances 2009; Fruchtnict 2010).

Where appropriate within the following categories and diagnoses of the DSM-IV, a **DSM-5** icon has been added to point out "potential" changes. Until the DSM-5 publishes, the DSM-IV-TR remains the appropriate current source for diagnostic categories and diagnoses (DSM5.org 2011; DSM-V 2009; Fox 2010). For ongoing updates, access www.DSM5.org.

Delirium, Dementia, and Amnestic Disorders

These disorders are characterized by clinically significant cognitive deficits and notable changes from previous levels of functioning. The changes may be due to a medical condition or substance abuse or both (APA 2000).

- **Dementia** – Characterized *by intellectual decline and usually progressive deficits* not only in memory but also in language, perception, learning, and other areas. *Dementia of the Alzheimer's type (AD) is the most common dementia,* followed by vascular dementia *(ischemic vascular dementia).* Other causes: Infections: HIV, encephalitis, Creutzfeldt-Jakob disease; drugs and alcohol (Wernicke-Korsakoff's syndrome [thiamine deficiency]); inherited such as Parkinson's disease and Huntington's disease. Some dementias (AD) are essentially irreversible and others potentially reversible (drug toxicities, folate deficiency).
  DSM-5 – Discussions include: Removing the term *Dementia* and subsuming Dementia of Alzheimer's type under overarching category such as Major Neurocognitive Disorders.
- **Delirium** – Organic brain syndrome resulting in a *disturbance in consciousness and cognition* that happens within a short period with a variable course.
- **Amnestic Disorder** – Disturbance in memory and impaired ability to learn new information or recall previously learned information.
- **Pseudodementia** – Cognitive difficulty that is caused by depression but may be mistaken for dementia. Need to consider and rule out in the elderly who may appear to have dementia when actually suffering from depression, which is a treatable disease. Could be depressed with cognitive deficits as well.

CLINICAL PEARL – AD is a progressive and irreversible dementia with a gradually declining course, whereas ischemic vascular dementia (ministrokes and transient ischemic attacks) often presents in a stepwise fashion with an acute decline in cognitive function. It is important to distinguish between dementia and delirium because delirium can be life-threatening and should be viewed as an emergency. Delirium can be differentiated from dementia by its *rapid onset, fluctuating in and out of a confusional state, and difficulty in attending to surroundings.* Delirium is usually caused by a physical condition, such as infection; therefore, the underlying cause needs to be treated. Keep in mind that a person with dementia may also become delirious.

Dementia of Alzheimer's Type (AD)

Signs & Symptoms	Causes	Rule Outs	Labs/Tests/Exams	Interventions
• Memory impairment • Inability to learn new material • Language deterioration (naming objects) • Inability to execute typical tasks (cook/ dress self) • Executive functioning disturbances (planning/abstract thinking/new tasks) • Paranoia • Progressive from mild forgetfulness to middle and late dementia (requiring total ADL care/ bedridden) • Course: 18 mo–27 y [avg. 10–12 y]	• Idiopathic • Many theories (viral/ trauma) • Pathology shows neuritic plaques and neurofibrillary tangles; also amyloid protein • Familial AD (presenilin 1 gene) • Apolipoprotein E genotype (Kukull 2002)	• Ischemic vascular dementia • Dementia with Lewy bodies • Alcoholic dementia (Wernicke-Korsakoff [thiamine deficiency]; pellagra [niacin deficiency]; hepatic encephalitis) • Delirium • Depression • Medical disorder (HIV, syphilis) • Other substance abuse • Psychosis	• Mental status exam • Folstein Mini-Mental State Exam • Neuropsychological testing (Boston naming; Wisconsin card sorting test) • Depression Rating Scales: D-ARK Scale; Beck (BDI); Geriatric Depression Scale (R/O depression) • CBC, blood chemistry (renal, metabolic/hepatic), sed rate, T4/TSH, B_{12}, folate, UA, FTA-Abs, CT scan/ MRI; HIV titer • **New:** Structural MRIs and CSF markers (continuing to investigate) (Andersson 2011; Vermuri 2010)	• Early diagnosis • Symptom treatment (aggression/ agitation) • Behavioral management • Communication techniques • Environmental safety checks • Antipsychotics • Antidepressants • Sedatives • Antianxiety agents • Nutritional supplements • Anti-Alzheimer's agents (e.g., donepezil [Aricept]); memantine (Namenda)

Dementia With Lewy Bodies

Clients with dementia with Lewy bodies usually present with pronounced changes in attention (drowsiness, staring), parkinsonian symptoms, and visual hallucinations; unlike AD, the course is usually rapid. Donepezil, rivastigmine, and levodopa may benefit cognitive/motor symptoms. Researchers are exploring newer methods for diagnosing and differentiating the dementias including CSF biomarkers (Andersson 2011) and structural MRI (Vermuri 2010).

◎ **ALERT**: Important to differentiate AD from dementia with Lewy bodies. Clients with Lewy bodies dementia are very sensitive to antipsychotics and, because of their psychosis (visual hallucinations), they are often treated with an antipsychotic. Such treatment often results in extrapyramidal symptoms (EPS) (Goroll 2009).

Early Diagnosis of Dementia

Mayo Clinic has developed a framework entitled STAND-Map (STructural Abnormality iNDex) in hopes of diagnosing dementia in living patients. Hopefully from this we will be able to differentiate among AD, Lewy Body disease, and frontotemporal lobe degeneration (Mayo Clinic 2009; Vermuri 2010).

Medications to Treat Dementia of the Alzheimer's Type

- Medications used to treat mild to moderate AD include tacrine [Cognex], donepezil [Aricept], rivastigmine (Exelon) and galantamine [Reminyl].
- Memantine (Namenda), which is an NMDA receptor antagonist, is the first drug approved for moderate to severe AD.
- Investigational drug: Amyloid deposit inhibitors: Clioquinoline may reduce amyloid deposits.

Client/Family Education: Dementia

- Educate family on how to **communicate with loved ones** with dementia, especially if paranoid. Family members should not argue with someone who is agitated or paranoid.
- Focus on positive behaviors, avoiding negative behaviors that do not pose a safety concern.
- Avoid arguments **by talking about how the dementia client is feeling rather than arguing the validity of a statement.** For instance, if the client says that people are coming into the house and stealing, family members can be taught to discuss the feelings around the statement rather than the reality of it ("That must be hard for you, and we will do all we can to keep you safe.").
- Educate family about **environmental safety,** as dementia clients may forget they have turned on a stove, or they may have problems with balance. Throw rugs may need to be removed and stove disconnected, with family members providing meals.

- Family members need to understand that this is a **long-term management issue requiring the support of multiple health professionals and family and friends.** Management may require medication (control of hostility or for hallucinations/delusions). Medications need to be started at low doses and titrated slowly.
- Keep in mind that a spouse or family caregiver is also dealing with his/her own feelings of loss, helplessness, and memories of the person who once was and no longer exists.
- Teach the family caregiver how to manage difficult behaviors and situations in a calm manner, which will help both the family member and the client.
- ***Caregiver stress.*** Remember that the caregiver also needs a break from the day-to-day stress of caring for someone with dementia. This could involve respite provided by other family members and friends (Chenitz et al 1991; WebMD Video 2010).

Substance-Related Disorders

- Substances include prescribed medications, alcohol, over-the-counter medications, caffeine, nicotine, steroids, illegal drugs, and others; substances serve as central nervous system (CNS) stimulants, CNS depressants, and pain relievers; and may alter both mood and behaviors.
- Many substances are accepted by society when used in moderation (alcohol, caffeine), and others are effective in chronic pain management (opioids) but can be abused in some instances and illegal when sold on the street.
- Substance use becomes a problem when there is recurrent and persistent use despite social, work, and/or legal consequences and despite a potential danger to self or others.

Substance Use Disorders

Substance Dependence

- Repeated use of drug despite substance-related cognitive, behavioral, and physiological problems.
- Tolerance, withdrawal, and compulsive drug-taking may result. There is a craving for the substance.
- Substance dependence does not apply to caffeine.

Substance Abuse

- Recurrent and persistent maladaptive pattern of substance use with significant adverse consequences occurring repeatedly or persistently during the same 12-month period.
- Repeated work absences, DUIs, spousal arguments, fights (APA 2000).

DSM-5 – Projected elimination of "substance abuse and dependence" as disease categories and replace with **Addictions and Related Disorders.** See DSM-5, Substance-Related Disorders, beginning of this tab.

Substance-Induced Disorders

Substance Intoxication

- Recent overuse of a substance, such as an acute alcohol intoxication, that results in a reversible, substance-specific syndrome.
- Important behavioral and psychological changes (alcohol: slurring of speech, poor coordination, impaired memory, stupor, or coma).
- Can happen with one-time use of substance.

Substance Withdrawal

- Symptoms differ and are specific to each substance (cocaine, alcohol).
- Symptoms develop when a substance is discontinued after frequent substance use (anxiety, irritability, restlessness, insomnia, fatigue) (APA 2000).

Addiction, Withdrawal, and Tolerance/Internet Addiction

- ***Addiction*** – The repeated, compulsive use of a substance that *continues in spite of negative consequences* (physical, social, legal, etc.).
  DSM-5 – Possible addition of "drug craving" as an addiction criteria.
- ***Physical Withdrawal/Withdrawal Syndrome*** – Physiological response to the abrupt cessation or drastic reduction in a substance used (usually) for a prolonged period. The symptoms of withdrawal are specific to the substance used.
- ***Tolerance*** – Increased amounts of a substance over time are needed to achieve the same effect as obtained previously with smaller doses/amounts.

See *Assessment Tab* for Screening Questionnaire, Short Michigan Alcohol Screening Test, and Substance History and Assessment.

- ***Internet Addiction*** – Even though there is no evidence or research suggesting Internet addiction exists as a disorder, behaviors can be compulsive, and the Internet offers many opportunities for sexual addicts. More research is needed (DeAngelis 2000; Ng & Weimer-Hastings 2005).

DSM-5 – A new category of addictions may be added, **Behavioral Addictions**, which includes "gambling." Internet addiction was considered but will likely be included in the Appendix until further research can be done.

Substance Dependence

Signs & Symptoms	Causes	Rule Outs	Labs/Tests/Exams	Interventions
• Maladaptive coping mechanism • Clinically significant impairment/ distress, same 12-mo period • Tolerance develops: increasingly larger amounts needed for same effect • Intense cravings and compulsive use; unsuccessful efforts to cut down • Inordinate time spent obtaining substance (protecting supply) • Important activities given up • Continue despite physical/ psychological problems	• Genetics (hereditary, esp. alcohol) • Biochemical • Psychosocial • Ethnocultural • Need to approach as biopsychosocial disorder • Response to substances can be very individualistic	• Consider comorbidities: mood disorders, such as bipolar/ depression. ECA study: (Reiger et al 1990) 60.7% diagnosed with bipolar I had lifetime diagnosis of substance use disorders • Untreated chronic pain • Undiagnosed depression in elderly (isolation a problem)	• SMAST, AUDIT, others • CAGE questionnaire • Toxicology screens (emergencies) • Arkansas-Depression (D-ARK) Scale; Beck Depression Inventory (BDI) (R/O depression) • GDS • Labs: Liver function tests (LFTs) – γ-glutamyltransferase (GGT) and mean corpuscular volume (MCV); % CDT (carbohydrate-deficient transferrin) (Anton 2001)	• Early identification and education • Confidential and nonjudgmental approach • Evaluate for comorbidities and treat other disorders • Evaluate own attitudes about substance use/ dependence • Psychotherapy • Behavior therapy • 12-step programs • Medications: mood stabilizers, antidepressants, naltrexone • Detoxification • Hospitalization

Client/Family Education: Substance-Related Disorders

- Keep in mind that most clients underestimate their substance use (especially alcohol consumption) and that denial is the usual defense mechanism.
- When substance dependence/abuse is suspected, it is important to approach the client in a supportive and nonjudgmental manner. Focus on the consequences of continued substance use and abuse (physically/emotionally/family/employment), and discuss the need for complete abstinence. Even with a desire to stop, there can be relapses.
- If a substance user/abuser will not seek help, then family members should be encouraged to seek help through organizations such as AlAnon (families of alcoholics) or NarAnon (families of narcotic addicts). AlaTeen is for adolescent children of alcoholics, and Adult Children of Alcoholics (ACOA) is for adults who grew up with alcoholic parents.
- For substance abusers, there is Alcoholics Anonymous, Narcotics Anonymous, Overeaters Anonymous, Smokers Anonymous, Women for Sobriety, etc. There is usually a support group available to deal with the unique issues of each addiction.
- In some instances, medication may be required to manage the withdrawal phase (physical dependence) of a substance. Benzodiazepines may be needed, including inpatient detoxification.
- Naltrexone, an opioid antagonist, reduces cravings by blocking opioid receptors in the brain and is used in heroin addiction and alcohol addiction (reduces cravings and number of drinking days) (Tai 2004; Rosner 2010).
- Educate clients and families about the possibility of comorbidities (bipolar disease) and the need to treat these disorders as well.

◎ **ALERT:** Be aware of the increase in *methamphetamine addiction* in North America, its highly addictive nature, and the devastating social and physical (neurotoxic) consequences of use (Barr et al 2006).

Schizophrenia and Other Psychotic Disorders

In 1908, *Eugen Bleuler,* a Swiss psychiatrist, introduced the term *schizophrenia,* which replaced the term dementia praecox, used by *Emil Kraepelin* (1896). Kraepelin viewed this disorder as a deteriorating organic disease; Bleuler viewed it as a serious disruption of the mind, a "splitting of the mind." In 1948, ***Fromm-Reichman*** coined the term ***schizophrenogenic mother,*** described as cold and domineering, although appearing self-sacrificing. ***Bateson*** (1973, 1979) introduced the ***double bind*** theory, wherein the child *could never win* and was always wrong (invalidation disguised as acceptance; illusion of choice; paradoxical communication).

- Schizophrenia ***is a complex disorder,*** and it is now accepted that schizophrenia is the result of neurobiological factors rather than due to some early psychological trauma.
  - The *lifetime prevalence rate* (US/worldwide) is about 1%.
  - Onset in the late teens to early 20s, equally affecting men and women.
  - Devastating disease for both the client and the family.
  - Schizophrenia affects thoughts and emotions to the point that social and occupational functioning is impaired (Susser 2006; Combs 2010).
  - About 9% to 13% of schizophrenics commit suicide (Meltzer 2003).
- ***Early diagnosis and treatment are critical*** to slowing the deterioration and decline, which will result without treatment. **DSM-5** – Considering adding "psychosis risk syndrome."

  ◎ **ALERT:** A new blood test, VeriPsych, is available to aid in the diagnosis of schizophrenia. This is a 51-biomarker test that may help with early onset schizophrenia diagnosis (Schwarz 2010; VeriPsych 2010).
  - Earlier typical antipsychotic drugs effective against most of the positive symptoms; less effective against negative symptoms.
  - Atypical antipsychotic drugs work on both negative and positive symptoms.
  - Family/community support is key factor in improvement.
- ***Subtypes of schizophrenia*** include paranoid, disorganized, catatonic, undifferentiated, and residual types. **DSM-5** – See DSM-5, Schizophrenia and other psychotic disorders, beginning of this tab, for deletions of these subtypes.
- ***National Association for the Mentally Ill*** (www.nami.org) is an important national organization that has done much to educate society and communities about mental illness and to advocate for the seriously mentally ill.
- ***Other psychotic disorders*** include schizophreniform disorder, schizoaffective disorder, delusional disorder, brief psychotic disorder, shared psychotic disorder (folie à deux), psychotic disorder due to a medical condition, substance-induced, and not otherwise specified (NOS).

Schizophrenia

Signs & Symptoms	Causes	Rule Outs	Labs/Tests/Exams	Interventions
• At least for 1 mo, two or more from the following: • Delusions • Hallucinations • Disorganized speech • Disorganized behavior • Negative symptoms (alogia, affective flattening, avolition) • Functional disturbances at school, work, self care, personal relations • Disturbance continues for 6 mo	• Dopamine hypothesis (excess) • Brain abnormalities (third ventricle sometimes larger) • Frontal lobe – decreased glucose use/smaller frontal lobe • Genetic – familial; monozygotic twin (47% risk vs 12% dizygotic) • Virus • No specific cause	• Schizophreniform disorder • Schizoaffective • Mood disorder with psychotic symptoms • Medical disorder/ substance abuse with psychotic episode • Delusional disorder • Note: with schizophrenia, the condition persists for at least 6 mo and is chronic and deteriorating	• Psychiatric evaluation and mental status exam • No test can diagnose schizophrenia • Positive and Negative Syndrome Scale (PANSS) • Abnormal Involuntary Movement Scale (AIMS) • Need to R/O other possible medical/ substance use disorders: LFTs, toxicology screens, CBC, thyroid function test (TFT), CT scan, etc. • **New**: VeriPsych blood test (measures 51 biomarkers) (Schwarz 2010; VeriPsych 2010)	• Antipsychotic – usually atypicals for new onset: olanzapine, aripiprazole, etc. • *New:* paliperidone (Invega) • Acute psychotic episode may need high potency (haloperidol) • Hospitalization until positive symptoms under control • Patient/family education • NAMI for patient/family education, patient advocate

Positive and Negative Symptoms of Schizophrenia

- **Positive Symptoms**

Positive symptoms are excesses in behavior (excessive function/ distortions)

  - Delusions
  - Hallucinations (auditory/visual)
  - Hostility
  - Disorganized thinking/behaviors

- **Negative Symptoms**

Negative symptoms are deficits in behavior (reduced function; self-care deficits)

  - Alogia
  - Affective blunting
  - Anhedonia
  - Asociality
  - Avolition
  - Apathy

Four A's of Schizophrenia

- Eugen Bleuler in 1911 proposed four basic diagnostic areas for characterizing schizophrenia. These became the 4 A's:
  A: Inappropriate **Affect**
  A: Loosening of **Associations**
  A: **Autistic** Thoughts
  A: **Ambivalence**
- These four A's provide a memory tool for recalling how schizophrenia affects thinking, mood (flat), thought processes, and decision-making ability (Shader 2003).

CLINICAL PEARL – When auditory hallucinations first begin, they usually sound soft and far away and eventually become louder. When the sounds become soft and distant again, the auditory hallucinations are usually abating. The majority of hallucinations in North America are auditory (versus visual), and it is unlikely that a client will experience both auditory and visual hallucinations at the same time.

Thought Disorders – Content of Thought (Definitions)

Common Delusions

Delusion of Grandeur – Exaggerated/unrealistic sense of importance, power, identity. Thinks he/she is the President or Jesus Christ.

Delusion of Persecution – Others are out to harm or persecute in some way. *May believe his/her food is being poisoned or he/she is being watched.*

Delusion of Reference – Everything in the environment is somehow related to the person. *A television news broadcast has a special message for this person solely.*

Somatic Delusion – An unrealistic belief about the body, such as *the brain is rotting away.*

Control Delusion – Someone or something is controlling the person. *Radio towers are transmitting thoughts and telling person what to do.*

Thought Disorders – Form of Thought (Definitions)

Circumstantiality – Excessive and irrelevant detail in descriptions with the person eventually making his/her point. *We went to a new restaurant. The waiter wore several earrings and seemed to walk with a limp...yes, we loved the restaurant.*

Concrete Thinking – Unable to abstract and speaks in concrete, literal terms. *For instance, a rolling stone gathers no moss would be interpreted literally.*

Clang Association – Association of words by sound rather than meaning. *She cried till she died but could not hide from the ride.*

Loose Association – A loose connection between thoughts that are often unrelated. *The bed was unmade. She went down the hill and rolled over to her good side. And the flowers were planted there.*

Tangentiality – Digressions in conversation from topic to topic and the person never makes his/her point. *Went to see Joe the other day. By the way, bought a new car. Mary hasn't been around lately.*

Neologism – Creation of a new word meaningful only to that person. *The hiphopmobilly is on its way.*

Word Salad – Combination of words that have no meaning or connection. *Inside outside blue market calling.*

Client/Family Education: Schizophrenia

- Client and family education is critical to improve chances of relapse prevention and to slow or prevent regression and associated long-term disability.
- Refer client/family to the National Association for the Mentally Ill (NAMI) (www.nami.org) (1-800-950-NAMI [6264]).

- Client needs both medication and family/community support.
- Studies have shown that clients taking medication can still relapse if living with high expressed emotion family members (spouse/parent). These family members are critical, intense, hostile, and overly involved versus low expressed emotion family members (Davies 1994).
- Once stabilized on medication, clients often stop taking their medication because they feel they no longer need their medication (denying the illness or believing they have recovered). It is important to stress the need for medication indefinitely and that maintenance medication is needed to prevent relapse.
- Clients also stop their medication because of untoward side effects. Engage the client in a discussion about medications so that he/she has some control about options. The newer atypical drugs have a better side-effect profile, but it is important *to listen to the client's concerns* (weight gain/EPS) as adjustments are possible or a switch to another medication. Educate client/family that periodic lab tests will be needed.

  ◎ **ALERT:** For those on antipsychotic therapy, there is also a concern with treatment-emergent diabetes, especially for those with risk factors for diabetes, such as family history, obesity, and glucose intolerance (Buse et al 2002; Smith 2008).
- Early diagnosis, early treatment, and ongoing antipsychotic maintenance therapy with family support are critical factors in slowing the progression of this disease and in keeping those with schizophrenia functional and useful members of society.

Mood Disorders

A mood disorder is related to a person's emotional tone or affective state and can have an effect on behavior and can influence a person's personality and worldview.

DSM-5 – Proposing an *anxiety dimension* across all mood disorders as well as a *suicide assessment dimension.*

- Extremes of mood (mania or depression) can have devastating consequences on client, family, and society alike.
- These consequences include financial, legal, marital, relationship, employment, and spiritual losses as well as despair that results in potential suicide and death.
- Correct diagnosis is needed, and effective treatments are available.

The **mood disorders** are divided into *depressive disorders* and *bipolar disorders.*

- The **depressive disorders** include major depressive disorder, dysthymic disorder, and depressive disorder NOS.
- The **bipolar disorders** include bipolar I disorder, bipolar II disorder, cyclothymic disorder, and bipolar disorder NOS.

Depressive Disorders

- **Major depressive disorder** (unipolar depression) requires at least 2 weeks of depression/loss of interest and four additional depressive symptoms, with one or more major depressive episodes.
- **Dysthymic disorder** is an ongoing low-grade depression of at least 2 years' duration for more days than not and does not meet the criteria for major depression.
- **Depression NOS** does not meet the criteria for major depression and other disorders (APA 2000).

Bipolar Disorders

- **Bipolar I disorder** includes one or more manic or mixed episodes, usually with a major depressive episode.
- **Bipolar II disorder** includes one or two major depressive episodes and at least one hypomanic (less than full mania) episode.
- **Cyclothymic disorder** includes at least 2 years of hypomanic periods that do not meet the criteria for the other disorders.
- **Bipolar NOS** does not meet any of the other bipolar criteria.
- **Others:** Mood disorders due to a general medical condition, substance-induced mood disorders, and mood disorder NOS (APA 2000).
  DSM-5 – Exploring how to better clarify boundary between unipolar depression and bipolar disorder.

*See **depression rating scales** (D-ARK, Geriatric) as well as **The Mood Disorder Questionnaire (MDQ)** (Hirschfeld 2003) for bipolar spectrum disorder in the Assessment Tab.*

SIGECAPS – Mnemonic for Depression

Following is a mnemonic for easy recall and review of the DSM-IV criteria for major depression or dysthymia:

Sleep (increase/decrease)
Interest (diminished)
Guilt/low self-esteem
Energy (poor/low)
Concentration (poor)

Continued

Appetite (increase/decrease)
Psychomotor (agitation/retardation)
Suicidal ideation

A depressed mood for 2 or more weeks, plus four SIGECAPS = major depressive disorder

A depressed mood, plus three SIGECAPS for 2 years, most days = dysthymia (Brigham and Women's Hospital 2001).

CLINICAL PEARL – Important to determine that a depressive episode is a unipolar depression versus a bipolar disorder *with a depressive episode.* A first-episode bipolar I or II may begin with major depression. The presentation is a "clinical snapshot in time" rather than the complete picture. Further evaluation and monitoring are needed. Bipolar clients are often misdiagnosed for years.

- One study (Ghaemi et al 2003) showed 37% of patients were misdiagnosed (depression vs bipolar), resulting in new or worsening rapid cycling (mania) in 23% because antidepressants were prescribed (Keck 2003).
- Although the tricyclic antidepressants (TCAs) are more likely to trigger a manic episode, the selective serotonin reuptake inhibitors (SSRIs) have also been implicated.
- **Postpartum Depression** – See Edinburgh Postnatal Depression Scale in Assessment Tab.

Postpartum Depression in Fathers

- Men can also develop postpartum depression with a 4%–25% chance. Three to six months showed the highest rate (25.6%). Twelve-month prevalence is 4.8% (Melrose 2010).
- Men need to be screened for depression, and depression in one parent warrants clinical attention to the other.
- Fathers should also be screened for depression using the EPDS with a cutoff score of over 10 (Edmondson 2010).

ALERT: If a client who is recently prescribed antidepressants begins showing manic symptoms, consider that this client may be bipolar.

Major Depressive Episode

Signs & Symptoms	Causes	Rule Outs	Labs/Tests/Exams	Interventions
• Depressed mood or loss of interest for at least 2 weeks and five or more of: • Significant weight loss/ gain • Insomnia or hypersomnia • Psychomotor agitation or retardation • Fatigue • Worthless feelings or inappropriate guilt • Problem concentrating • Recurrent thoughts of death	• Familial predisposition (female to male, 3:1) • Deficiency of norepinephrine (NE) and serotonin • Hypothalamic dysfunction • Psychosocial factors • Unknown	• Bipolar I or II disorder • Schizoaffective • Grief (major loss) (acute distress → 3 mo) • Postpartum depression • Thyroid/adrenal dysfunction; hypothyroidism • Neoplasms • CNS (stroke) • Vitamin deficiencies (folic acid) • Medication (reserpine, prednisone) • Pseudodementia (older adult) • Substance abuse disorder (cocaine)	• Psychiatric evaluation and mental status exam • D-ARK Scale (see Assessment Tab); BDI; Zung Self-Rating Depression Scale; Geriatric Depression Scale • Mood Disorder Questionnaire (MDQ) • MMSE • Physical exam • R/O other possible medical/ substance use disorders: LFTs, toxicology screens, CBC, TFT, CT scan, etc.	• Antidepressants: usually SSRIs (fluoxetine, sertraline); selective norepinephrine reuptake inhibitors (SNRIs) (venlafaxine) • *TCAs:* side effects include sedation, dry mouth, blurred vision; TCAs not good for elderly (falls) • MAOIs • *New:* selegiline patch (Emsam) • Others: bupropion • Cognitive behavioral therapy (CBT) • Psychotherapy • Electroconvulsive therapy (ECT) • *Emerging:* • Vagal nerve stimulation • Transcranial magnetic stimulation

Manic Episode

Signs & Symptoms	Causes	Rule Outs	Labs/Tests/Exams	Interventions
• Persistent elevated, irritable mood ≥1 wk, plus three or more (irritable, four or more): • ↑ Self-esteem • ↓ Sleep • ↑ Talk/pressured speech • Racing thoughts/ flight of ideas • Distractibility • Extreme goal-directed activity • Excessive buying/ sex/business investments (painful consequences)	• Genetic: familial predisposition (female to male, 1.2:1) • Bipolar onset 18–20 yr • Catecholamines: NE, dopamine • Many hypotheses: serotonin, acetylcholine; neuroanatomical (frontotemporal lesions) • Complex disorder	• Hypomanic episode (bipolar II) • Mixed episode (major depressive and manic episode ≥1 wk) • Cyclothymia • Substance-induced (cocaine) • ADHD • Dual diagnosis • Brain lesion • General medical condition	• Psychiatric evaluation and mental status exam • Young Mania Rating Scale (YMRS) (bipolar I) • Mood Disorder Questionnaire • Need to R/O other possible medical/ substance use/ induced disorders: LFTs, toxicology screens, CBC, TFT, CT scan, etc.	• Mood stabilizers: lithium (standard); anticonvulsants (carbamazepine, valproic acid, lamotrigine, topiramate) • Combined treatments: lithium and anticonvulsant • Antipsychotics: e.g., aripiprazole, olanzapine • Lithium: + for mania/not for mixed • Therapy and medication compliance

Postpartum Major Depressive Episode

Signs & Symptoms	Causes	Rule Outs	Labs/Tests/Exams	Interventions
• Symptoms similar to major depressive episode • Acute onset to slowly over first 3 postpartum (PP) months • Persistent/ debilitating vs blues • Depressed mood, tearfulness, insomnia, suicidal thoughts • Anxiety, obsession about well-being of infant • Affects functioning	• Occurs in 10%–15% of women and in men, 4%–25% • Highest risk: hx of depression, previous PP depression, depression during pregnancy • Previous PP depression with psychosis: ↑ 30%–50% risk of recurrence at subsequent delivery	• PP blues: (fluctuating mood; peaks 4th d post delivery; ends 2 weeks; functioning intact) • PP psychosis: 1 – 2/1000 women; ↑ risk: bipolar/previous PP psychosis; infanticide/ suicide risk high • Medical cause	• Edinburgh Postnatal Depression Scale (EPDS): self-rated questionnaire (see Assessment Tab); also to screen fathers • Screen during PP period • Psychiatric evaluation • Physical exam • Routine lab tests: CBC, TFT (thyroid/ anemia)	• Pharmacological: SSRIs, SNRIs, TCAs (insomnia); consider weight gain, dry mouth, sedation with TCAs • CBT, individual, group psychotherapy • Anxiolytics • ECT • Psychosis: hospitalization; mood stabilizers, antipsychotics, ECT

Client/Family Education: Mood Disorders

Mood disorders can range from subthreshold to mild (dysthymic) to extreme (manic/psychotic) fluctuations in emotion and behaviors.

Family and client need educating about the specific disorder, whether major depression, bipolar I or II, postpartum depression, or unresolved grief. Without treatment, support, and education, the results can be devastating emotionally, interpersonally, legally, and financially.

- The mood disorders need to be explained in terms of their biochemical basis – "depression is an illness, not a weakness," although often recurrent, chronic illness.
- Families and clients need to understand that early diagnosis and treatment are essential for effective management and improved outcome.
- It may be helpful to compare with other chronic illnesses, such as diabetes and asthma, as a model and to reinforce the biological basis of the illness to reduce stigma. As with any chronic illness (diabetes, asthma), ongoing management, including pharmacological treatment, is required, realizing there may be exacerbations and remissions.
- Reinforce the need to adhere to the dosing schedule as prescribed and not to make any unilateral decisions, including stopping, without conferring with health professional.
- Work with client and family on side-effect management. If client can be part of the decision making when there are options, client will be more willing to become involved in own recovery and continue treatment.
- Address weight gain possibilities (lithium, anticonvulsants, antipsychotics); monitor weight, BMI, exercise, and food plans to prevent weight gain.
- Other treatment options for depression: Mindfulness CBT and transcranial magnetic stimulation (Segal 2010; George 2010).

Anxiety Disorders

- The anxiety disorders include a wide range of disorders from the very specific, such as phobias, to generalized anxiety disorder, which is pervasive and experienced as dread or apprehension.
- Other anxiety disorders include panic disorder, agoraphobia (avoidance of places that may result in panic), social phobia, obsessive-compulsive disorder, posttraumatic stress disorder, acute stress disorder, anxiety due to a medical disorder, substance-induced anxiety disorder, and anxiety disorder NOS.
- Some anxiety is good, motivating people to perform at their best. Excessive anxiety can be crippling and may result in the "fight or flight" reaction. The fighter is ever ready for some perceived aggression and is unable to relax, and the escaper (flight) freezes with anxiety and may avoid upsetting situations or actually dissociate (leave his/her body/fragment).

- Either extreme is not good and can result in physical and emotional exhaustion. (See Fight-or-Flight Response and Stress-Adaptation Syndrome in Basics Tab.)

  DSM-5 – PTSD – "Developmental manifestations" being developed as age-specific criteria to make diagnoses across all age groups. "Anxiety dimensions" proposed for all mood disorders.

Four Levels of Anxiety

- *Mild Anxiety* – This is the anxiety that can motivate someone positively to perform at a high level. It helps a person to focus on the situation at hand. For instance, this kind of anxiety is often experienced by performers before entering the stage.
- *Moderate Anxiety* – Anxiety moves up a notch with narrowing of the perceptual field. The person has trouble attending to his/her surroundings, although he/she can follow commands/direction.
- *Severe Anxiety* – Increasing anxiety brings the person to another level, resulting in an inability to attend to his/her surroundings, except for maybe a detail. Physical symptoms may develop, such as sweating and palpitations (pounding heart). Anxiety relief is the goal.
- *Panic Anxiety* – The level reached is now terror, where the only concern is to escape. Communication impossible at this point (Peplau 1963).

CLINICAL PEARL – Recognizing level of anxiety is important in determining intervention. Important to manage anxiety before it escalates. At the moderate level, firm, short, direct commands are needed: *You need to sit down, Mr. Jones.*

DSM-5 – *Obsessive-compulsive disorder may be reclassified under "anxiety and obsessive-compulsive spectrum disorders." "Body dysmorphic disorder" (currently a somatoform disorder) may also move to this new classification.*

Obsessive-Compulsive Disorder (OCD)

Signs & Symptoms	Causes	Rule Outs	Labs/Tests/Exams	Interventions
• *Obsessions* – recurrent, intrusive thoughts that cause anxiety OR *Compulsions* – repetitive behaviors (hand washing, checking) that reduce distress/anxiety and must be adhered to rigidly • Driven to perform compulsions • Time-consuming (>1 hr/d), interfere with normal routine • Recognizes thoughts/behaviors are unreasonable	• Genetic evidence • Neurobiological basis: orbitofrontal cortex, cingulate, and caudate nucleus • Neurochemical: serotonergic and possibly dopaminergic • Association between OCD and Tourette's, and others • Lifetime prevalence of 2.5% • Women > men • Avg onset: 20 y • Childhood: 7–10 y	• Other anxiety disorders: phobias • Impulse control disorders • Obsessive-compulsive personality disorder • Body dysmorphic disorder • Depression • Neurological disorders	• Yale-Brown Obsessive-Compulsive Scale (Y-BOCS) • Psychiatric evaluation • Mental status exam • Neurological exam	• Pharmacological: SSRIs: fluoxetine: (higher doses); fluvoxamine; clomipramine • Beta blockers: propranolol • Behavior therapy: exposure and response prevention • Deep muscle relaxation • Individual and family therapy • Education

Generalized Anxiety Disorder (GAD)

Signs & Symptoms	Causes	Rule Outs	Labs/Tests/Exams	Interventions

• Excessive anxiety; at least 6 mo; difficult to control worry/ hypervigilant
• Associated with three or more:
  • Restless/on edge
  • Easily fatigued
  • Concentration problems
  • Irritability
  • Muscle tension
  • Sleep disturbance
  • Causes significant distress
  • Often physical complaints: dizziness, tachycardia, tightness of chest, sweating, tremor
	• Neurotransmitter dysregulation: NE, 5-HT, GABA
	• Autonomic nervous system activation: locus ceruleus/NE release/limbic system
	• 1-year prevalence rate: 1%; lifetime prevalence, 5%
	• Familial association
	• Over half: onset in childhood
		• Anxiety disorder due to a medical condition (hyperthyroidism; pheochromocytoma)
		• Substance-induced anxiety or caffeine-induced anxiety disorder
		• Other anxiety disorders: panic disorder, OCD, etc.; DSM-IV criteria help rule out
			• Self-rated scales: Beck Anxiety Inventory (BAI); State Trait Anxiety Inventory
			• Observer-rated scale: Hamilton Anxiety Rating Scale (HAM-A)
			• Psychiatric evaluation
			• Physical exam
			• Routine lab tests; TFTs
				• Pharmacological: benzodiazepines very effective (diazepam, lorazepam); non-benzodiazepines: buspirone
				• Antidepressants, (SSRIs): escitalopram and paroxetine
				• Beta blockers: propranolol
				• CBT
				• Deep muscle relaxation
				• Individual and family therapy
				• Education

Posttraumatic Stress Disorder (PTSD)

Signs & Symptoms	Causes	Rule Outs	Labs/Tests/Exams	Interventions
• Traumatic event (self/family/ witness others); threat of harm or death or actual death and helplessness • Reexperiencing event "flashbacks" (triggers: sounds/ smell) • Hypervigilance/ recurrent nightmares/ numbing • Anniversary re-actions (unaware reenactment re-lated to trauma) • Persistent anxiety/ outbursts • Acute (<3 mo); chronic (≥3 mo); delayed (>6 mo)	• Rape, torture, child abuse, natural disaster, murder, war, terrorism, etc. • Physiological/ neurochemical/ endocrinological alterations • Sympathetic hyperarousal • Limbic system (amygdala dysfunction) • "Kindling": ↑ neuronal excitability • Risk factor: previous trauma • Combat military 3-fold increase since 2001 • Lifetime preva-lence ~8% (US)	• Acute stress disorder • Obsessive-compulsive disorder • Adjustment disorder • Depression • Panic disorder • Psychotic disorders • Substance-induced disorder • Psychotic disorder due to a general medical condition • Delirium	• PTSD scale (clinician-administered) • PTSD checklist, civilian version (Weathers 1991) • Psychiatric evaluation • Mental status exam • Neurological exam • CAGE, SMAST • Physical exam, routine blood studies • No laboratory test can diagnose	• Debriefing (rescuers, etc.) • Individual or group psychotherapy • CBT • Eye Movement Desensitization and Reprocessing (EMDR) (Shapiro 2001) • Pharmacotherapy: Antidepressants – SSRIs, SNRIs, MAOIs, TCAs; antipsychotics; anxiolytics; mood stabilizers • Family and community support/art therapy/ psychodrama

Client/Family Education: Anxiety Disorders

Anxiety, the most common disorder in the United States, exists along a continuum and may be in response to a specific stressor (taking a test), or it may present as a generalized "free-floating" anxiety (GAD) or a panic disorder (PD) (feeling of terror). A 1-year prevalence rate for all anxieties has been said to be about 18.1% (NIMH 2010).

- Most people have experienced some degree of anxiety, so it might be helpful for family members to understand the four stages of anxiety and how one stage builds on the other – especially in trying to explain panic disorder.
- It is important for families to understand the importance of early diagnosis and treatment of anxiety disorders, as these are chronic illnesses and will become worse and more difficult to treat over time.
- Explain to client and family the need for ongoing management (pharmacological/education/psychotherapeutic/CBT), *just as diabetes, asthma, and heart disease must be managed.*
- Many of these disorders are frustrating to family members. It is hard to understand the repetitive hand washing or checking that can be done by someone with OCD. Family members are also affected, and the client's illness becomes a family issue as well.
- The client may also need to be educated about the needs of other family members (maybe time away from client [respite]). Family therapy may be needed to negotiate and agree on living arrangements in a way that respects the needs of the client and all family members.
- As in all chronic disorders, remissions and exacerbations will be experienced. At times reinforcement sessions (CBT) are needed, especially with CBT and exposure/response prevention for OCD.
- Remind families that patience, persistence, and a multimodal/multiteam approach to treatment are needed.

Somatoform Disorders

Somatoform disorders are characterized by physical symptoms that suggest a physical disorder, but are not fully explained by a general medical condition. Following is a listing of somatoform disorders:

- **Somatization Disorder** (see table that follows) begins before age 30 with multiple symptoms (pain, GI, sexual, and pseudoneurological), lasting a long time (years).
  DSM-5 – Somatization disorder may be subsumed under "complex somatic symptom disorders."

- **Undifferentiated Somatoform Disorder** is similar to somatization disorder but does not qualify for somatization disorder (less intense/not as pronounced/less impairment), and symptoms last at least 6 months.
- **Conversion Disorder** affects voluntary motor/sensory functions, which causes significant distress or impairment socially or in other areas of functioning, but cannot be explained by a medical/neurological condition.
- **Pain Disorder** – the focus of attention is pain itself of sufficient severity to warrant clinical attention, with psychological factors playing a key role.
- **Hypochondriasis** involves fear of disease and idea that one has a serious disease, despite medical evidence to the contrary, and a focus on the body's symptoms/functions for at least 6 months.
- **Body Dysmorphic Disorder (BDD)** is an obsession/preoccupation with an (perceived) exaggerated "defect" (nose, lips, eyes) in physical appearance, with frequent checking in the mirror. Preoccupation causes significant distress or social, occupational, or other functional impairment.
  DSM-5 – BDD may possibly be reclassified in "anxiety and obsessive-compulsive spectrum disorders."
- **Somatoform Disorder NOS** – Does not meet criteria for any of the somatoform disorders (APA 2000).

Somatization Disorder (SD)

Signs & Symptoms	Causes	Rule Outs	Labs/Tests/Exams	Interventions

• Hx of physical complaints before age 30 over several years; seeking Rx or affects important areas of functioning
• Each must be met:
  • Four pain symptoms in four different areas (head/back/stomach/joint pain)
  • Two GI symptoms (N, V)
  • One sexual symptom (ED, pain)
  • One pseudoneurological symptom (paralysis/balance)
  • Cannot be fully explained by a medical condition or a substance OR physical symptoms are in excess of history/lab findings
  • Symptoms are not feigned
	• Prevalence rates of 0.2%–2% for women and less than 0.2% for men
	• Observed in 10% – 20% of female first degree relatives with SD
	• Male relatives of women with SD have increased risk of antisocial personality disorder and substance-related disorders
	• May be underlying mood disorder
		• Somatoform disorder NOS (symptoms <6 mo)
		• General medical condition
		• Schizophrenia
		• Panic disorder
		• Depressive disorder
		• Anxiety disorder
		• Factitious disorder
		• Malingering
		• Pain disorder associated with...
			• Psychiatric evaluation
			• Mental status exam
			• Neurological exam
			• Physical exam, routine blood studies
			• No lab test is remarkable for these subjective complaints
			• Must R/O medical condition
				• Antidepressants
				• Stress management
				• Lifestyle changes (exercise)
				• Collaboration between primary care physician and mental health provider (MHP)
				• Psychotherapy
				• CBT
				• Psychoeducation
				• Family support
				• Support/understanding – client often believes symptoms are physical/refuses psychological help
				• Avoid unnecessary medical treatments/tests (often doctor/hospital shops)
				• Chronic fluctuating disorder – rarely remits

Sexual and Gender Identity Disorders

The Sexual and Gender Identity Disorders are divided into three main categories by the DSM-IV-TR. In order to understand dysfunction, sexual health needs to be defined and understood.

- ***Sexual health*** is defined as a state of physical, emotional, mental, and social well-being related to sexuality; it is not merely the absence of disease or dysfunction. It requires a respectful and positive approach, free of coercion, discrimination, and violence. Sexual practices are safe and have the possibility of pleasure (WHO 1975).
- A person's ***sex*** refers to *biological* characteristics that define this person as a male or a female (some individuals possess both male and female biological characteristics [hermaphrodite/intersex]) (WHO 2002).
- ***Gender*** refers to the characteristics of men and women that are *socially constructed* rather than biologically determined. People are taught the *behaviors* and *roles* that result in their becoming men and women, also known as *gender identity* and *gender roles.*
  - Gender roles are also culturally determined and differ from one culture to another; they are not static; they are also affected by the law and religious practice.
  - Gender also relates to power relationships (between men and women) as well as reproductive rights issues and responsibilities (APA 2000).
- ***Sexual orientation*** refers to the sexual preference of a person, whether male to female, female to female, male to male, or bisexual. Variations in sexual preference are considered to be sexually healthy (APA 2000).

Sexual Dysfunctions

- *Sexual dysfunction* is a disturbance in the sexual response cycle or is associated with pain during intercourse.
- ***Sexual response cycle dysfunctions*** include the areas of desire, excitement, orgasm, and resolution. Categories include: hypoactive sexual desire disorder, sexual aversion disorder, female sexual arousal disorder, male erectile disorder, female and male orgasmic disorders, and premature ejaculation. **DSM-5** – Addition: "hypersexual disorder" and deletion: "sexual aversion disorder."
- The *pain disorders* include: dyspareunia, vaginismus, sexual function due to a medical disorder, substance-induced sexual dysfunction, and sexual dysfunction NOS.

Paraphilias

- The *paraphilias* are sexually arousing fantasies, urges, or behaviors triggered by/focused on nonhuman objects, self or partner humiliation, nonconsenting adults, or children, which are recurrent for a period of at least 6 months.
- There are episodic paraphilias that operate only during times of stress.
- ***Paraphilias*** include *pedophilia* (sexual activity with a child ≤13 y); *frotteurism* (touching/rubbing nonconsenting person); *fetishism* (nonhuman object used for/needed for arousal); *exhibitionism* (genital exposure to a stranger); *voyeurism* (observing unsuspecting persons naked or in sexual activity); *sexual masochism* (humiliation/suffering), *sadism* (excitement from inflicting suffering/humiliation); and others (APA 2000).

Gender Identity Disorder

- Gender Identity Disorder requires a cross-gender *identification* and a belief and insistence that "one is the other sex." The desire is persistent, and the preference is for cross-sex roles. Prefers the stereotypical roles and games/pastimes/clothing of other sex.
- There exists an extreme and persistent discomfort with the biological sex at birth and the sense of oneself as not belonging to the gender role of the biological sex.
- Boys will have an aversion to own penis and testicles, and girls resent growing breasts or female clothing.
- This is not a physical intersex condition, and there is definite distress over the biological sex that affects important areas of functioning (APA 2000).

DSM-5 – *Gender identity disorder* may be changed to *gender incongruence* to better reflect the core issue.

Because sexuality and its dysfunctions involve cultural considerations and attitudes, moral and ethical concerns, religious beliefs, as well as legal considerations, it is important to evaluate your own beliefs, values, possible prejudices, and comfort level in dealing with sexual disorders.

Hypoactive Sexual Desire Disorder

Signs & Symptoms	Causes	Rule Outs	Labs/Tests/Exams	Interventions
• Deficiency or absence of sexual fantasies or desires; persistent/recurrent • Marked distress/interpersonal difficulties • Not substance-induced or due to a general medical condition • Does not usually initiate sex and reluctantly engages in sex with partner • Relationship/marital difficulties • Lifelong/acquired/situational	• Psychological: partner incompatibility, anger, sexual identity issues, sexual preference issues, negative parental views (as a child)	• Sexual aversion disorder (intense fear/disgust over sex vs disinterest) • Extremes in sexual appetite (sexual addict as a partner) • Major depression • Medical condition • Substance abuse • Medication • Sexual abuse • Other	• Complete physical exam, including medical history • Psychiatric evaluation • Mental status exam • Sexual history • Routine lab work, thyroid function tests • BDI • D-ARK Scale • Zung • CAGE • SMAST	• Refer to sex therapist • Relationship therapy • CBT • Assuming no physical/medication/substance use disorder, deal with relationship issues and assure sexual compatibility and sexual orientation • **DSM-5** – This disorder may be subsumed under new disorder "sexual interest/arousal disorder"

Client/Family Education: Sexual/Gender Identity Dysfunctions/Paraphilias/Gender Identity Disorders

Sexual Dysfunctions

- Clients and their partners need to understand where in the sexual response cycle the problem exists (arousal/orgasm).
- If the problem is one of desire or aversion, this needs to be explored further to determine the causes: couple discord, gender identity, sexual orientation issues, negative views of sexual activity, previous sexual abuse, body image, or self-esteem issues.
- The same holds true for other sexual dysfunctions (orgasmic problems/erectile dysfunction) in that issues around substance use/abuse; previous sexual experiences; possible psychological, physical, and other stressors as factors, including medical conditions and prescribed medications, need to be explored.
- Referral to a sex therapist may be needed to find ways to reconnect intimately. Sometimes partner education is needed on how to satisfy the other partner (mutual satisfaction).

Paraphilias and Gender Identity Disorders

The Paraphilias and Gender Identity Disorders require help from professionals especially trained in dealing with these disorders. Clients and families need to receive support and education from these professionals.

Eating Disorders

- Eating disorders are influenced by many factors, including family rituals and values around food and eating, ethnic and cultural influences, societal influences, and individual biology.
- American society currently stresses physical beauty and fitness and favors the thin and slim female as the ideal.
- There has been a dramatic increase in the number of obese people in the United States – at an alarming rate among children.
- With society's emphasis on fast and convenient foods, high in calories, a reduction in exercise (computers/TV), and the ongoing value of "thin as beautiful," eating disorders remain a concern.

  DSM-5 – Renaming as "eating and feeding disorders." Add binge eating disorder.

Anorexia Nervosa/Bulimia Nervosa

- Two specific eating disorders are anorexia nervosa (AN) and bulimia nervosa (BN). *(For BN see table that follows.)* Both use/manipulate eating behaviors in an effort to control weight. Each has its dangers and consequences if maintained over time.
- ***Anorexia Nervosa*** – The AN client is terrified of gaining weight and does not maintain a minimally acceptable body weight.
  - There is a definite disturbance in the perception of the size or shape of the body.
  - AN is more common in the industrialized societies and can begin as early as age 13 y.
  - Body weight in the anorexic client is less than 85% of what would be expected for that age and height.
  - Even though underweight, client still fears becoming overweight.
  - Self-esteem and self-evaluation based on weight and body shape.
  - Amenorrhea develops, as defined by absence of three consecutive menstrual cycles (APA 2000).

Client/Family Education: Eating Disorders

- Client and family need to understand the serious nature of both disorders; mortality rate for AN clients is 2%–8% (30%–40% recover; 25%–30% improve; 15%–20% do not improve). About 50% of BN clients recover with treatment (Rakel 2000).
- *Team approach important* – client and family need to be involved with the team, which should or may include a nutritionist, psychiatrist, therapist, physician, psychiatric nurse, nurse, eating disorder specialist, and others.
- Teach client coping strategies, allow for expression of feelings, teach relaxation techniques, and help with ways (other than food) to feel in control.
- Family therapy important to work out parent-child issues, especially around control (should have experience with eating disorders).
- Focus on the fact that clients do recover and improve, and encourage patience when there is a behavioral setback.

Bulimia Nervosa (BN)

Signs & Symptoms	Causes	Rule Outs	Labs/Tests/Exams	Interventions
• Recurrent binge eating of large amount of food over short period • Lack of control and cannot stop • Self-induced vomiting, laxatives (purging), fasting, exercise (nonpurging) to compensate • At least 2 ×/w for 3 mo • Normal weight; some underweight/overweight • Tooth enamel erosion/ finger or pharynx bruising • Fluid & electrolyte disturbances	• Genetic predisposition • Hypothalamic dysfunction implication • Family hx of mood disorders and obesity • Issues of power and control • Societal emphasis on thin • Affects 1%–3% women • Develops late adolescence through adulthood	• Anorexia nervosa, binge-eating, purging type • Major depressive disorder (MDD) with atypical features • BPD • General medical conditions: Kleine-Levin syndrome • Endocrine disorders	• Complete physical exam • Psychiatric evaluation • Mental status exam • Routine lab work, including TFT, CBC, electrolytes, UA • D-ARK Scale; BDI • MDQ • ECG • SMAST • CAGE	• Individual, group, marital, family therapy • Behavior modification • Nutritional support • Medical support • Client-family education

Personality Disorders

- When a pattern of relating to and perceiving the world is inflexible and maladaptive, it is described as a personality disorder.
- The pattern is enduring and crosses a broad range of social, occupational, and personal areas.
- The pattern can be traced back to adolescence or early adulthood and may affect cognition, affect, interpersonal functioning, or impulse control.

DSM-5 – The personality disorders will be reformulated and use a "dimensional view" of PDs. Will focus on types, traits, facets, severity level, and a new definition.

Cluster A Personality Disorders

- Cluster A disorders include the paranoid personality, schizoid personality, and schizotypal personality disorders.
- This cluster includes the distrustful, emotionally detached, eccentric personalities.

Cluster B Personality Disorders

- Cluster B disorders include the antisocial, borderline (BPD), histrionic, and narcissistic personality disorders. **DSM-5** – Discussions of making BPD an Axis I disorder. May also rename as borderline type with type and trait ratings (severity scales).
- This cluster includes those who have disregard for others, with unstable and intense interpersonal relationships, excessive attention seeking, and entitlement issues with a lack of empathy for others.

Cluster C Personality Disorders

- Cluster C personality disorders include the avoidant personality, dependent personality, and the obsessive-compulsive personality disorders.
- This cluster includes the avoider of social situations; the clinging, submissive personality; and the person preoccupied with details, rules, and order (APA 2000).

Borderline Personality Disorder (BPD)

Signs & Symptoms	Causes	Rule Outs	Labs/Tests/Exams	Interventions
• Pattern of unstable interpersonal relationships • Fear of abandonment • Splitting: idealize and devalue (love/hate) • Impulsive (four areas: sex, substance abuse, binge eating, reckless driving) • Suicidal gestures/ self-mutilation • Intense mood changes lasting a few hours • Chronic emptiness • Intense anger • Transient paranoid ideation	• Genetic predisposition • Family hx of mood disorders; may be a variant of/related to bipolar disorder • Physical/ sexual abuse • About 2% of general population • Predominantly female (75%)	• Mood disorders (often co-occur) • Histrionic, schizotypal, paranoid, antisocial, dependent, and narcissistic PDs • Personality change due to a general medical condition	• Millon Clinical Multiaxial Inventory-III (MCMI-III) • Psychiatric evaluation • Mental status exam • D-ARK Scale; BDI • CAGE • SMAST • Physical exam, routine lab work, TFT	• Linehan (1993) dialectical behavior therapy (DBT) • CBT • Group, individual, family therapy (long-term therapy) • Special strategies • Boundary setting • Be aware that these can be difficult clients even for experienced MH professionals • Pharmacotherapy: antidepressants, mood stabilizers, antipsychotics; caution with benzodiazepines (dependence)

Client/Family Education: Personality Disorders

- Share personality disorder with client and family and educate about the disorder. In this way the client has a basis/framework to understand his/her recurrent patterns of behavior.
- Work with client and family in identifying most troublesome behaviors (temper tantrums), and work with client on alternative responses and to anticipate triggers.
- For clients who act out using suicidal gestures, an agreement may have to be prepared that helps client work on impulse control. Agreement might set an amount of time that client will not mutilate and what client will do instead (call a friend/therapist/listen to music). Need to teach alternative behaviors.
- It is better to lead clients to a conclusion *("Can you see why your friend was angry when you did such and such?")* rather than tell the client what he or she did, especially those clients with a BPD.
- Because these are long-standing, fixed views of the world, they require time and patience and can be frustrating to treat. Usually require an experienced therapist.
- Although BPD receives much attention, all clients with personality disorders (narcissist, dependent, avoidant personalities) suffer in relationships, occupations, social situations.
- Client needs to be willing to change, and a therapeutic (trusting) relationship is a prerequisite for anyone with a personality disorder to accept criticisms/frustrations. Some clients believe the problems rest with everyone but themselves.
- Helpful books for BPD clients and families to read in order to understand the borderline personality include: Kreisman JJ, Straus H: *I Hate You – Don't Leave Me.* [rev], Perigee, 2010, and Kreisman JJ, Straus H: *Sometimes I Act Crazy: Living with Borderline Personality Disorder.* Hoboken, NJ, John Wiley & Sons, 2006.
- For professionals: Linehan MM. *Skills Training Manual for Treating Borderline Personality Disorder.* New York: Guilford Press, 1993, and Linehan MM. *Cognitive-Behavioral Treatment of Borderline Personality Disorder.* New York: Guilford Press, 1993.

Disorders of Childhood and Adolescence

Disorders diagnosed in childhood or adolescence include:

- Mental retardation – onset before age 18 and IQ <70.
  DSM-5 – Mental retardation to change to "intellectual disability."
- Learning disorders – include mathematics, reading disorder; disorder of written expression, with academic functioning below age, education level, intelligence.

- Communication disorders – speech or language difficulties, including expressive language, mixed receptive-expressive language, phonological disorder, and stuttering.
- Motor skills – developmental coordination disorder, with poor motor coordination for age and intelligence.
- Pervasive developmental disorders – deficits in multiple developmental areas, including autism, Asperger's, Rett's, and childhood disintegrative disorder.
  DSM-5 – Rett's possibly removed; Asperger's included in new category: Autism spectrum disorders.
- Feeding/eating disorders – disturbances of infancy and childhood, including pica, rumination, and feeding disorder of infancy and early childhood.
  DSM-5 – Reclassification of pica and feeding disorders (move to Eating and Feeding Disorders).
- Tic disorders – vocal and motor tics such as Tourette's, transient tic, and chronic motor or vocal tic disorder.
- Elimination disorders – include encopresis and enuresis.
- Attention deficit/disruptive behavior – includes ADHD, predominantly inattentive, predominantly hyperactive-impulsive, or combined type; conduct disorder, oppositional defiant disorder, and others.
- Others – separation anxiety, selective mutism, reactive attachment disorder, and so forth (APA 2000).

Mental Retardation	
50 – 70 IQ MILD	Able to live independently with some assistance; some social skills; does well in structured environment
35 – 49 IQ MODERATE	Some independent functioning; needs to be supervised; some unskilled vocational abilities (workshop)
20 – 34 IQ SEVERE	Total supervision; some basic skills (simple repetitive tasks)
<20 IQ PROFOUND	Total care and supervision; care is constant and continual; little to no speech/no social skills ability

Modified from Townsend 5th ed., 2010, with permission

Attention Deficit/Hyperactivity Disorder (ADHD)

- ADHD is characterized either by *persistent inattention* or by *hyperactivity/impulsivity* for at least 6 months.
- Inattention includes:
  - Carelessness and inattention to detail
  - Cannot sustain attention and does not appear to be listening
  - Does not follow through on instructions and unable to finish tasks, chores, homework
  - Difficulty with organization and dislikes activities that require concentration and sustained effort
  - Loses things; distracted by extraneous stimuli; forgetful
- Hyperactivity-impulsivity includes:
  - Hyperactivity
  - Fidgeting, moving feet, squirming
  - Leaves seat before excused
  - Runs about/climbs excessively
  - Difficulty playing quietly
  - "On the go" and "driven by motor"
  - Excessive talking

DSM-5 – Inattentive/hyperactive/impulsive, a minimum of 4 symptoms if a person is 17 y or older.

- Impulsivity
  - Blurts out answers, speaks before thinking
  - Problem waiting his/her turn
  - Interrupts or intrudes
- Impairment is present before age 7 y, and impairment is present in at least two settings (or more). **DSM-5** – Proposes presence of symptoms by age 12 y.
- Significant impairment in functioning in social, occupational, or academic setting. Symptoms are not caused by another disorder. Prevalence rate, school-aged children: 3%–7% (APA 2000).
- Many *possible* causes: genetics; biochemical (possible neurochemical deficits [dopamine, NE]); intrauterine exposure to substances such as alcohol or smoking; exposure to lead, dyes, and additives in food; stressful home environments.
- Adult ADHD – Study presented at American Psychiatric Association on the prevalence in the US (Farone 2004); ADHD estimated at 4.1% in adults, ages 18–44, in a given year (NIMH 2010).

Nonpharmacological ADHD Treatments

- Individual/family therapy
- *Behavior modification:* clear expectations and limits

- Break commands up into clear steps
- Support desired behaviors and immediately respond to undesired behaviors with consequences
- *Natural consequences* helpful (loses bicycle; do not replace; has to save own money to replace)
- *Time outs* may be needed for cooling down/reflecting
- *Role playing:* helpful in teaching friend-friend interactions; helps child prepare for interactions and understand how intrusive behaviors annoy and drive friends away
- *Inform school:* important that school knows about ADHD diagnosis, as this is a disability (Americans With Disabilities Act)
- Seek out special *education services*
- *Classroom:* sit near teacher, one assignment at a time, written instructions, untimed tests, tutoring (need to work closely with teacher and explain child's condition [ADHD])
- *Nutritional:* many theories remain controversial but include food sensitivities (Feingold diet, allergen elimination, leaky gut syndrome, Nambudripad's allergy elimination technique), supplementation (thiamine), minerals (magnesium, iron), essential fatty acids, amino acids; evaluate for lead poisoning

For Pharmacological ADHD Treatments – *See Drugs/Labs Tab.*

Conduct Disorder/Oppositional Defiant Disorder

- *Conduct disorder (CD)* (serious rule violation, aggression, destruction) and *oppositional defiant disorder (ODD)* (negative, hostile, defiant) are other important disorders of childhood and adolescence.
  DSM-5 – Proposing addition of "temper dysregulation disorder" to better differentiate from bipolar disorder and ODD.
- Serious comorbidities include CD/ADHD, ODD/ADHD, and CD/ADHD/GAD/MDD.
- A position paper by the International Society of Psychiatric-Mental Health Nurses, entitled *Prevention of Youth Violence,* can be found at: http://ispn-psych.org/docs/3-01-youth-violence.pdf

---

Because of size limitations, PsychNotes *can provide only limited and basic information related to the unique and comprehensive specialty of child and adolescent psychiatry. For more complete coverage, refer to any of the standard psychiatric textbooks and references.*

Psychiatric Interventions

Therapeutic Relationship/Alliance

- The *therapeutic relationship* is not concerned with the skills of the mental health professional (MHP) but rather with the attitudes and the relationship between the MHP and the client. This relationship comes out of the creation of a safe environment, conducive to communication and trust.
- An *alliance* is formed when the professional and the client are working together cooperatively in the best interest of the client. The therapeutic relationship begins the moment the MHP and client first meet (Shea 1999).

Core Elements of a Therapeutic Relationship

- Communication/rapport – It is important to establish a connection before a relationship can develop. Encouraging the client to speak, using open-ended questions, is helpful. Asking general (not personal) questions can relax the client in an initial session. It is important to project a caring, nonjudgmental attitude.
- *Trust* – A *core element of a therapeutic relationship.* Many clients have experienced disappointment and unstable, even abusive, relationships. Trust develops over time and remains part of the process. *Without trust, a therapeutic relationship is not possible.* Other important elements are *confidentiality, setting boundaries, and consistency.*
- *Dignity/Respect* – Many clients have been abused and humiliated and have low self-esteem. If treated with dignity through the therapeutic relationship, clients can learn to regain their dignity.
- *Empathy* – Empathy is not sympathy (caught up in client's feelings) but is, rather, open to understanding the "client's perceptions" and helps the client understand these better through therapeutic exploration.
- *Genuineness* – Genuineness relates to trust because it says to the client: *I am honest, and I am a real person.* Again, it will allow the client to get in touch with her/his "real" feelings and to learn from and grow from the relationship.

Therapeutic Use of Self

Ability to use one's own personality consciously and in full awareness to establish relatedness and to structure interventions (Travelbee 1971). Requires self-awareness and self-understanding.

Phases of Relationship Development

- *Orientation phase* – This is the phase when the MHP and client *first meet* and *initial impressions are formed.*
  - Rapport is established, and trust begins.

- The relationship and the connection are most important.
- Client is encouraged to identify the problem(s) and become a collaborative partner in helping self.
- Once rapport and a connection are established, the relationship is ready for the next phase.

- *Identification phase* – In this phase the MHP and client are:
  - Clarifying perceptions and setting expectations in and for the relationship.
  - Getting to know and understand each other.
- *Exploitation (working) phase* – The client is committed to the process and to the relationship and is involved in own self-help; takes responsibility and shows some independence.
  - This is known as the *working phase* because this is when the hard work begins.
  - Client must believe and know that the MHP is caring and *on his/her side* when dealing with the more difficult issues during therapeutic exploration.
  - *If this phase is entered too early,* before trust is developed, clients may suddenly terminate if presented with painful information.
- *Resolution phase* – The client has gained all that he/she needs from the relationship and is ready to leave.
  - This may involve having met stated goals or resolution of a crisis.
  - Be aware of fear of abandonment and need for closure.
  - Both the MHP and client may experience sadness, which is normal.
  - Dependent personalities may need help with termination, reflecting upon the positives and the growth that has taken place through the relationship (Peplau 1992).
- If a situation brings a client back for therapy, the relationship has already been established (trust); therefore, *there is not a return to the orientation phase.* Both will identify new issues and re-establish expectations of proposed outcomes. It will now be *easier to move into the working phase of the relationship,* and this will be done more quickly.

CLINICAL PEARL – *Trust* and *safety* are core elements of a therapeutic alliance, as many clients have experienced abuse, inconsistency, broken promises, and "walking on eggs."

Nonverbal Communication

Nonverbal communication may be a better indication of what is going on with a client than verbal explanations.

- Although verbal communication is important, it is only one component of an evaluation.
- Equally important to develop your skills of observation.
- Some clients are not in touch with their feelings, and only their behaviors (clenched fist, head down, arms crossed) will offer clues to feelings.

- Nonverbal communication may offer the client clues as to how the MHP is feeling as well.
- *Physical appearance* – A neat appearance is suggestive of someone who cares for him/herself and feels positive about self. Clients with schizophrenia or depression may appear disheveled and unkempt.
- *Body movement/posture* – Slow or rapid movements can suggest depression or mania; a slumped posture, depression. Medication-induced body movements and postures include: pseudoparkinsonism (antipsychotic); akathisia (restlessness/moving legs [antipsychotic]). Warmth (smiling) and coldness (crossed arms) are also nonverbally communicated.
- *Touch* – Touch forms a bridge or connection to another. Touch has different meanings based on culture, and some cultures touch more than others. Touch can have a very positive effect, but touching requires permission to do so. Many psychiatric clients have had "boundary violations," so an innocent touch may be misinterpreted.
- *Eyes* – The ability to maintain eye contact during conversation offers clues as to social skills and self-esteem. Without eye contact, there s a "break in the connection" between two people. A lack of eye ontact can suggest suspiciousness, something to hide. Remember cultural interpretations of eye contact (see Basics Tab).
- *Voice* – Voice can be a clue to the mood of a client. Pitch, loudness, and rate of speech are important clues. Manic clients speak loudly, rapidly, and with pressured speech. Anxious clients may speak with a high pitch and rapidly. Depressed clients speak slowly, and obtaining information may feel like "pulling teeth."

Communication Techniques

Technique	Rationale	Example
Reflecting	Reflects back to clients their emotions, using their own words	C: *John never helps with the housework.* MHP: *You're angry that John doesn't help.*
Silence	Allows client to explore all thoughts/feelings; prevents cutting conversation at a critical point or missing something important	MHP nods with some vocal cues from time to time so C knows MHP is listening but does not interject.

Continued

Communication Techniques—cont'd

Technique	Rationale	Example
Paraphrasing	Restating, using different words to ensure you have understood the client; helps clarify	C: *My grandkids are coming over today and I don't feel well.* MHP: *Your grandkids are coming over,* but you wish they weren't, *because you are not well. Is that what you are saying?*
Making observations	Helps client recognize feelings he/she may not be aware of and connect with behaviors	MHP: *Every time we talk about your father* you become very sad.
Open-ended/ broad questions	Encourages client to take responsibility for direction of session; avoids yes/no responses	MHP: *What would you like to deal with in this session?*
Encouragement	Encourages client to continue	MHP: *Tell me more...uh huh...and then?*
Reframing	Presenting same information from another perspective (more positive)	C: *I lost my keys, couldn't find the report, and barely made it in time to turn my report in.* MHP: *In spite of all that,* you did turn your report in.
Challenging idea/ belief system	Break through denial or fixed belief; always done with a question	MHP: *Who told you that you were incompetent? Where did you get the idea that you can't say no?*
Recognizing change/ recognition	Reinforces interest in client and positive reinforcement (this is not a compliment)	MHP: *I noticed that you were able to start our session today rather than just sit there.*
Clarification	Assures that MHP did not misunderstand; encourages further exploration	MHP: *This is what I thought you said...; is that correct?*

Continued

Communication Techniques—cont'd

Technique	Rationale	Example
Exploring in detail	If it appears a particular topic is important, then the MHP asks for more detail; MHP takes the lead from the client (client may resist exploring further)	MHP: *This is the first time I've heard you talk about your sister; would you like to tell me more about her?*
Focusing	Use when a client is covering multiple topics rapidly (bipolar/anxious) and needs help focusing	MHP: *A lot is going on, but* let's discuss the issue of your job loss, *as I would like to hear more about that.*
Metaphors/ symbols	Sometimes clients speak in symbolic ways and need translation	C: *The sky is just so gray today and night comes so early now.* MHP: *Sounds like you are feeling somber.*
Acceptance	Positive regard and open to communication	MHP: *I hear what you are saying. Yes, uh-huh* (full attention).

Therapeutic Milieu*

- In the therapeutic milieu (*milieu* is French for surroundings or environment), the entire environment of the hospital is set up so that every action, function, and encounter is therapeutic.
- The therapeutic community is a smaller representation of the larger community/society outside.
- The coping skills and learned behaviors within the community will also translate to the larger outside community.

Seven Basic Assumptions:

1. The health in each individual is to be realized and encouraged to grow.
2. Every interaction is an opportunity for therapeutic intervention.
3. The client owns his or her own environment.

4. Each client owns his or her own behavior.
5. Peer pressure is a useful and powerful tool.
6. Inappropriate behaviors are dealt with as they occur.
7. Restrictions and punishment are to be avoided (Skinner 1979).

*Difficult in era of managed care (short stays).

Group Interventions

Stages of Group Development

I. Initial Stage (in/out)

- Leader orients the group and sets the ground rules, including confidentiality.
- There may be confusion and questions about the purpose of the group.
- Members question themselves in relation to others and how they will fit in the group.

II. Conflict Stage (top/bottom)

- Group is concerned with pecking order, role, and place in group.
- There can be criticism and judgment.
- Therapist may be criticized as group finds its way.

III. Cohesiveness (Working) Stage (near/far)

- After conflict comes a group spirit, and a bond and trust develop among the members.
- Concern is now with closeness, and an "us versus them" attitude develops: those in the group versus those *outside the group.*
- Eventually becomes a mature working group.

IV. Termination

- Difficult for long-term groups; discuss well before termination.
- There will be grieving and loss (Yalom 2005).

Leadership Styles

- **Autocratic** – The autocratic leader essentially "rules the roost." He or she is the most important person of the team and has very strong opinions of how and when things should be done. Members of a group are not allowed to make independent decisions, as the autocrat trusts only his/her opinions. The autocrat is concerned with power and control and is very good at persuasion. High productivity/low morale.
- **Democratic** – The democratic leader focuses on the group and empowers the group to take responsibility and make decisions. Problem solving and taking action are important, along with offering alternative solutions to problems (by group members). Lower productivity/high morale.

- **Laissez-Faire** – This leaderless style results in confusion because of the lack of direction and noninvolvement; it also results in low productivity and morale (Lippitt & White 1958).

Individual Roles/Difficult Group Members

- **Monopolizer** – Involved in some way in every conversation, offering extensive detail or always presents with a "crisis of the week" (minimizing anyone else's concerns/issues).
  - Has always experienced a similar situation: I know what you mean; my dog died several years ago, and it was so painful I am still not over it.
  - Will eventually cause anger and resentment in the group if leader does not control the situation; dropouts result.
- **Help-rejecting complainer** – Requests help from the group and then rejects each and every possible solution so as to demonstrate the hopelessness of the situation.
  - No one else's situation is as bad as that of the help-rejecting complainer. *(You think you have it bad; wait until you hear my story!)*
  - Often looks to the group leader for advice and help and competes with others for this help, and because he/she is not happy, no one else can be happy either.
- **Silent client** – Does not participate but observes.
  - Could be fear of self-disclosure, exposing weaknesses. Possibly feels unsafe in leaderless group.
  - Does not respond well to pressure or being put on the spot, but must somehow be respectfully included and addressed.
  - The long-term silent client does not benefit from being in a group, nor does the group, and should possibly withdraw from the group.
- **Boring client** – No spontaneity, no fun, no opinions, and a need to present to the world what the client believes the world wants to see and hear.
  - If you are bored by the client, likely the client is boring.
  - Requires the gradual removal of barriers that have kept the individual buried inside for years.
  - Often tolerated by others but seldom missed if leaves the group.
- **Narcissist** – Lack of awareness of others in the group; seeing others as mere appendages and existing for one's own end; feels special and not part of the group (masses).
  - Expects from others but gives nothing.
  - Can gain from some groups and leaders.
- **Psychotic client** – Should not be included in early formative stages of a group.
  - If a client who is a member of an established group decompensates, then the group can be supportive because of an earlier connection and knowledge of the nonpsychotic state of the person.

- **Borderline client** – Can be challenging in a group because of emotional volatility, unstable interpersonal relationships, fears of abandonment, anger control issues, to name a few.
  - Borderline clients idealize or devalue (splitting) – the leader is at first great and then awful.
  - Some borderline group members who connect with a group may be helped as trust develops and borderline client is able to accept some frustrations and mild criticisms (Yalom 2005).

CLINICAL PEARL – It is important to understand that subgroups (splitting off of smaller group/unit) can and do develop within the larger group. Loyalty transferred to a subgroup undermines overall goals of larger group (some clients are in and some out). May be indirect hostility to leader. Some subgroups and extragroup activities are positive as long as there is not a splintering from/hostility toward larger group. Group needs to openly address feelings about subgroups and outside activities – if splintering or secretiveness continues, will be a detriment to group's cohesiveness and therapeutic benefit.

Yalom's Therapeutic Factors

The factors involved in and derived from the group experience that help and are of value to group members and therapeutic success are:

- *Instillation of hope* – Hope that this group experience will be therapeutic and effective.
- *Universality* – Despite individual uniqueness, there are common denominators that allow for a connection and reduce feelings of being alone in one's plight.
- *Didactic interaction* – In some instances, instruction and education can help people understand their circumstances, and such information relieves anxiety and offers power, such as understanding cancer, bipolar disorder, or HIV.
- *Direct advice* – In some groups, advice giving can be helpful when one has more experience and can truly help another (cancer survivor helping newly diagnosed cancer patient). Too much advice giving can impede. Advice giving/talking/refusing tells much about the group members and stage of group.
- *Altruism* – Although altruism suggests a concern for others that is unselfish, it is learning that through giving to others, one truly receives. One can find meaning through giving.
- *Corrective recapitulation of the primary family group* – Many clients develop dysfunctions related to the primary group – *the family of origin.* There are often unresolved relationships, strong emotions, and unfinished business. The group often serves as an opportunity to work out some of these issues as leaders and group members remind each other of primary family members, even if not consciously.

- *Socializing techniques* – Direct or indirect learning of social skills. Helpful to those whose interpersonal relationships have fallen short because of poor social skills. Often provided by group feedback, such as *You always turn your body away from me when I talk and you seem bored.* In many instances, individuals are *unaware* of the behaviors that are disconcerting or annoying to others.
- *Imitative behavior* – Members may model other group members, which may help in exploring new behaviors.

Family Therapy

Family Therapy Models/Theories

- *Intergenerational* – The theory of Murray Bowen (1994) that states problems are multigenerational and pass down from generation to generation until addressed. Requires direct discussion and clarification with previous generation members if possible. Concerned with level of individual differentiation and anxiety, triangles, nuclear family emotional system, and multigenerational emotional process. Therapist must remain a neutral third party.
- *Contextual* – The therapy of *Boszormenyi-Nagy* that focuses on give and take between family members, entitlement and fulfillment, fairness, and the family ledger (an accounting of debits and merits).
- *Structural* – Developed by *Salvador Minuchin* and views the family as a social organization with a structure and distinct patterns. Therapist takes an active role and challenges the existing order.
- *Strategic* – Associated with *Jay Haley* and focuses on problem definition and resolution, using active intervention.
- *Communications* – Focuses on communications in the family and emphasizes reciprocal affection and love; the *Satir model.*
- *Systemic* – Involves multidimensional thinking and use of paradox (tactics that appear opposite to therapy goals but designed to achieve goals); also called the *Milan model.*

CLINICAL PEARL – In dealing with families, it is important to have an understanding of how families operate, whatever model is used. A model offers a framework for viewing the family. A family is a subsystem within a larger system (community/society) and will reflect the values and culture of that society. Unlike working with individuals, it is the *family that is the client.*

Genogram

A genogram is a visual diagram of a family over two or three generations. It provides an overview of the family and any significant emotional and medical issues and discord among members. It offers insight into patterns and unresolved issues/conflicts throughout the generations.

Common Genogram Symbols

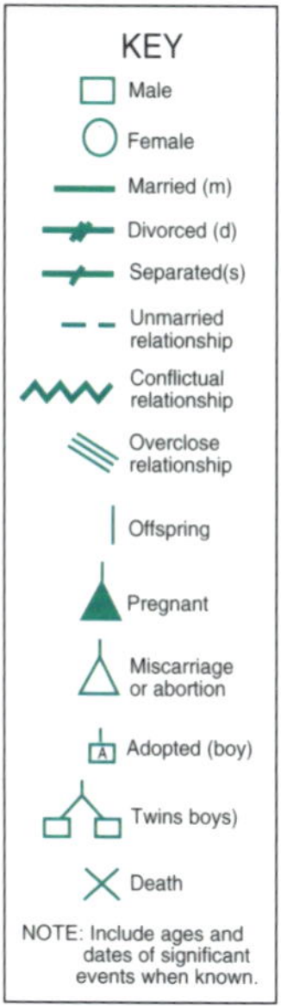

From Townsend 5th ed., 2010, with permission.

Sample Genogram

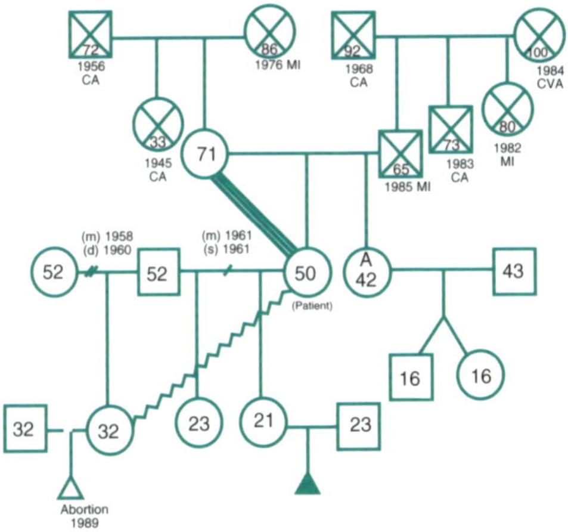

From Townsend 5th ed., 2010, with permission.

Cognitive Behavioral Therapy

- Cognitive behavioral therapy (CBT) deals with the relationship between cognition, emotion, and behavior.
  - Cognitive aspects are: automatic thoughts, assumptions, and distortions.
  - Individuals are often unaware of the *automatic thoughts* that may affect beliefs and behaviors, such as *I never do well in school* or *I am stupid.*
  - Deep-seated beliefs, or *schemas,* affect perceptions of the world.
  - Individuals are also influenced by *distortions* in their thinking.
- Important aspects of CBT include agenda setting, review, feedback, and homework.
- Some techniques may involve treating the behaviors rather than the cognitive aspects.
  - Fearful, dysfunctional clients respond better to behavioral versus cognitive interventions. This may involve task or activity assignments.

- Other behavioral interventions are: social skills training, assertiveness training, deep-muscle relaxation, exposure and systematic desensitization techniques, and in vivo interventions (phobias/agoraphobia). (Freeman et al 2004)

Distortions in Thinking

- *Catastrophizing* – an uncomfortable event is turned into a catastrophe.
- *Dichotomous thinking* – *either/or thinking,* such as *I am good* or *I am evil.*
- *Mind reading* – believes that the person knows what the other is thinking without clarifying.
- *Selective abstraction* – focusing on one aspect rather than all aspects. Individual hears only the one negative comment during a critique and does not hear the five positive comments.
- *Fortune telling* – anticipates a negative future event without facts or outcome. *I know I am going to fail that test.*
- *Overgeneralization* – one event is now representative of the entire situation. A forgotten anniversary is interpreted as: the marriage is over and will never be the same.

Mindfulness-Based Cognitive Therapy (MBCT)

MBCT is proving effective in the treatment of recurrent MDD. Mindfulness is an open, accepting, nonjudgmental awareness of self "in the present" and has proved very effective when combined with CBT (Segal 2010).

CLINICAL PEARL – CBT has been shown to be quite effective in treating depression and anxiety disorders (panic/phobia/OCD) and is very helpful when used in conjunction with medication. Through CBT, clients learn to change their thinking and to "reframe" their views/thoughts as well as learn tools/techniques to deal with future episodes. CBT provides the client with a sense of control over his/her fears, depression, and anxiety, as there is an active participation in treatment and outcome. Mindfulness CBT is proving even more effective in some instances, especially depression (Segal 2010).

Emerging/New Nonpharmacological Treatments for Depression

- Novel treatments are emerging in the treatment of depression, some showing clinical benefit and needing further study.
  - **Vagal nerve stimulation** – uses a small implantable device and is indicated for the adjunctive long-term treatment of chronic or recurrent depression for patients 18 years of age or older who are experiencing a major depressive episode and have not had an adequate response to four or more adequate antidepressant treatments (Cyberonics Inc. 2007; Nemeroff et al 2006).
  - **Transcranial magnetic stimulation** – noninvasive, relatively painless novel technique to alter brain physiology (Rachid & Bertschy 2006). Recent study has shown statistically significant and meaningful antidepressant effect especially in treatment-resistant depression (George 2010).

Complementary Therapies

- *Art therapy* – the use of art media, images, and the creative process to reflect human personality, interests, concerns, and conflicts. Very helpful with children and traumatic memories.
- *Biofeedback* – learned control of the body's physiological responses either voluntarily (muscles) or involuntarily (autonomic nervous system), such as the control of blood pressure or heart rate.
- *Dance therapy* – as the mind/body is connected, dance therapy focuses on direct expression of emotion through the body, affecting feelings, thoughts, and the physical and behavioral responses.
- *Guided imagery* – imagination is used to visualize improved health; has positive effect on physiological responses.
- *Meditation* – self-directed relaxation of body and mind; health-producing benefits through stress reduction. *See Mindfulness-based cognitive therapy.*
- *Others:* humor therapy, deep-muscle relaxation, prayer, acupressure, Rolfing, pet therapy, massage therapy, and so forth.

CLINICAL PEARL – Never underestimate the benefit of the complementary therapies. Complementary is often referred to as alternative therapy. In some ways, alternative is a misnomer because these are not alternatives but should be complements to traditional treatments. Both go hand in hand in a comprehensive approach to healing and treatment of the body, mind, and spiritual self.

Eye Movement Desensitization and Reprocessing (EMDR)

Developed by Francine Shapiro and involves therapist-directed rapid eye movements that are simultaneously associated with distressing or traumatic thoughts/memories. Bilateral brain stimulation (when eyes are rapidly moved from side to side) helps "reprocess" memories to relieve distress. This has been shown to be an effective treatment for PTSD (Shapiro 2001).

Psychotropic Drugs/Labs

Psychotropic Drugs

Labs/Plasma Levels

Psychotropic Drugs

Therapeutic Drug Classes

Antianxiety (Anxiolytic) Agents

Used in the treatment of generalized anxiety, obsessive-compulsive disorder (OCD), posttraumatic stress disorder (PTSD), phobic disorders, insomnia, and others and include:

- Benzodiazepines (alprazolam, clonazepam, lorazepam, oxazepam)
- Azaspirone (buspirone)
- Alpha-2 adrenergics (clonidine)
- Antihistamines (hydroxyzine)
- Beta blockers (propranolol)
- Antidepressants (doxepin, escitalopram)
- Hypnosedatives for insomnia, such as barbiturates (phenobarbital) and imidazopyridine (zolpidem)

Antidepressant Agents

Used in the treatment of depression, bipolar (depressed), OCD, and others, and include:

- Tricyclics (amitriptyline, desipramine, doxepin, imipramine)
- Monoamine oxidase inhibitors (MAOIs) (phenelzine, tranylcypromine)
- Selective serotonin reuptake inhibitors (SSRIs) (fluoxetine, paroxetine, sertraline)
- Serotonin norepinephrine reuptake inhibitors (SNRIs) (venlafaxine, duloxetine)
- Others (aminoketone/triazolopyridine) (bupropion [Wellbutrin], trazodone [Desyrel])

Mood-Stabilizing Agents

Used in the treatment of bipolar disorder (mania/depression), aggression, schizoaffective, and others, and include:

- Lithium
- Anticonvulsants (valproic acid, carbamazepine, lamotrigine, topiramate)
- Calcium channel blockers (verapamil)
- Alpha-2 adrenergics (clonidine) and beta adrenergics (propranolol)

Antipsychotic (Neuroleptic) Agents

Used in the treatment of schizophrenia, psychotic episodes (depression/organic [dementia]/substance-induced), bipolar disorder, agitation, delusional disorder, and others, and include:

- Conventional antipsychotics:
  - phenothiazines (chlorpromazine, thioridazine)
  - butyrophenones (haloperidol)
  - thioxanthenes (thiothixene)
  - diphenylbutyl piperidines (pimozide)

- dibenzoxazepine (loxapine)
- dyhydroindolone (molindone)

- Atypical antipsychotics:
  - dibenzodiazepine (clozapine)
  - benzisoxazole (risperidone)
  - thienobenzodiazepine (olanzapine)
  - benzothiazolyl piperazine (ziprasidone)
  - dihydrocarbostyril (aripiprazole)
  - dibenzo-oxepino pyrroles (asenapine)
  - piperidinyl-benzisoxazole (iloperidone)

(Modified from Pedersen: Pocket Psych Drugs 2010)

Although other agents (e.g., stimulants) may be used in the treatment of psychiatric disorders, the most common therapeutic classes and agents are listed above.

Pharmacokinetics

- *The Cytochrome P-450 Enzyme System* is involved in drug biotransformation and metabolism. It is important to develop a knowledge of this system to understand drug metabolism and especially drug interactions. Over 30 P-450 isoenzymes have been identified. The major isoenzymes include CYP1A2/2A6/2B6/2C8/2C9/2C18/2C19/2D6/2E1/3A4/3A5-7.

  Half-Life is the time (hours) that it takes for 50% of a drug to be eliminated from the body. Time to total elimination involves halving the remaining 50%, and so forth, until total elimination. Half-life is considered in determining dosing frequency and time to steady state. The rule of thumb for **steady state** (stable concentration/manufacture effect) **attainment** is 4–5 half-lives. *Because of fluoxetine's long half-life, a 5-week washout is recommended after stopping fluoxetine and before starting an MAOI to avoid a serious and possibly fatal reaction.*

  Protein Binding is the amount of drug that binds to the blood's plasma proteins; the remainder circulates unbound. It is important to understand this concept when prescribing two or more highly protein-bound drugs as one drug may be displaced, causing increased blood levels and adverse effects.

Antipsychotics and Treatment-Emergent Diabetes

Clients receiving atypical antipsychotics (especially clozapine and olanzapine) and also some conventional antipsychotics are at risk for developing diabetes and metabolic syndrome. Many atypicals are being prescribed for adjunctive treatment of depression as well as bipolar disorder. It is critical to monitor weight, BMI, FBS, as well as waist circumference in an effort to anticipate, prevent, and manage these possibilities (Nielsen 2010).

Body Mass Index (BMI)

The intersection of your weight and height equals your BMI. A BMI greater than 30 puts clients at greatest risk for cardiovascular disease/diabetes and other disorders. The preferred BMI is between 19 and 24. Risk increases between 25 and 29 (National Institutes of Health: Clinical Guidelines on the Identification, Evaluation, and Treatment of Overweight and Obesity in Adults: The Evidence Report, September 1998).

Metabolic Syndrome

Metabolic syndrome is defined as a group of clinical symptoms/criteria including abdominal obesity, hypertension, and diabetes, as well as low HDL (high density lipoprotein) levels and high levels of triglycerides. There is now a greater concern about the development of metabolic syndrome for those prescribed antipsychotics (Remington 2006). It is important to monitor waist circumference, BMI, weight, blood pressure, lipids, fasting blood sugar, and Hgb A1C, if diabetic.

Waist circumference should be <40 inches (102 cm) for men and <35 inches (88 cm) for women.

Clinical Identification of the Metabolic Syndrome

Any three of the following:

Risk Factor	Defining Level
Abdominal obesity Men Women	Waist circumference >102 cm (>40 in) >88 cm (>35 in)
Triglycerides	>150 mg/dL
HDL cholesterol Men Women	 <40 mg/dL <50 mg/dL
Blood pressure	>130/>85 mmHg
Fasting glucose	>110 mg/dL

Source: National Institutes of Health. ATP III Guidelines, National Cholesterol Education Program, NIH Publication No. 01-3305.
From Pedersen: Pocket Psych Drugs 2010, with permission.

Attention Deficit Hyperactivity Disorder (ADHD) Agents

Chemical Class	Generic/Trade	Dosage Range/Day
Amphetamines	Dextroamphetamine sulfate (Dexadrine)	5–60 mg
	Methamphetamine (Desoxyn)	5–25 mg
Amphetamine mixtures	Dextroamphetamine/ amphetamine (Adderall)	5–60 mg
Miscellaneous	Methylphenidate (Ritalin; Methylin; Concerta; Metadate)	10–60 mg
	Dexmethylphenidate (Focalin)	5–20 mg
	Pemoline (Cylert)	37.5–112.5 mg
	Atomoxetine (Strattera)	>70 kg: 40–100 mg; ≤70 kg: 0.5–1.4 mg/kg
	Bupropion (Wellbutrin)	3 mg/kg

From Townsend 2009; Pedersen 2010. Used with permission.

Antidepressants in Childhood and Adolescence

ALERT: Childhood depression has been on the rise in the United States, coupled with an increase in the prescribing of antidepressants for adolescents and also for children under age 5. In 2003, in the UK, suicidality in children was linked to Seroxat (Paxil), and now all antidepressants are linked to the possibility of increased suicidality in children and adolescents as well as young adults. Clearly, all children treated with antidepressants, as well as adults, need to be closely monitored (face to face), especially early in treatment, and assessed for suicidal ideation and risk (Johnson 2003; Seroxat 2004; Health Canada 2004).

Antiparkinsonian Agents

These are *anticholinergics* used to treat drug-induced parkinsonism, Parkinson's disease, and extrapyramidal symptoms (EPS). These include:

- Benztropine (Cogentin)
- Biperiden (Akineton)
- Trihexyphenidyl (Artane)
- Amantadine (dopaminergic) and diphenhydramine (antihistaminic) and others

Anticholinergic side effects include:

- Blurred vision, dry mouth, constipation
- Sedation, urinary retention, tachycardia

ALERT: Use cautiously in the elderly and in cardiac arrhythmias.

Antipsychotic Use Contraindications

- Addison's disease
- Bone marrow depression
- Glaucoma (narrow angle)
- Myasthenia gravis

Antipsychotic-Induced Movement Disorders

Extrapyramidal Symptoms (EPS)

EPS are caused by antipsychotic treatment and need to be monitored/evaluated for early intervention.

- Akinesia – rigidity and bradykinesia
- Akathisia – restlessness; movement of body; unable to keep still; movement of feet (do not confuse with anxiety)
- Dystonia – spasmodic and painful spasm of muscle (torticollis [head pulled to one side])
- Oculogyric crisis – eyes roll back toward the head. This is an emergency situation.
- Pseudoparkinsonism – simulates Parkinson's disease with shuffling gait, drooling, muscular rigidity, and tremor
- Rabbit syndrome – rapid movement of the lips that simulate a rabbit's mouth movements

Tardive Dyskinesia

Permanent dysfunction of voluntary muscles. Affects the mouth – tongue protrudes, smacking of lips, mouth movements.

ALERT: Evaluate clients on antipsychotics for possible tardive dyskinesia by using the Abnormal Involuntary Movement Scale (AIMS) (see AIMS form in Assessment Tab).

Drug-Herbal Interactions

Antidepressants should not be used concurrently with: St. John's wort or SAMe (serotonin syndrome and/or altered antidepressant metabolism).

Benzodiazepines/sedative/hypnotics should not be used concurrently with chamomile, skullcap, valerian, or kava. St. John's wort may reduce the effectiveness of benzodiazepines metabolized by P450 CYP3A4.

Conventional antipsychotics (haloperidol, chlorpromazine) that are sedating should not be used in conjunction with chamomile, skullcap, valerian, or kava. Carbamazepine, clozapine, and olanzapine should not be used concurrently with St. John's wort (altered drug metabolism/effectiveness).

ALERT: Ask all clients specifically what, if any, herbal or OTC medications they are using to treat symptoms.

Elderly and Medications (Start Low, Go Slow)

- Relevant drug guides provide data about dosing for the elderly and debilitated clients; also see Drugs A-Z Tab.
- The elderly or debilitated clients are started at lower doses, often half the recommended adult dose. This is due to:
  - Decreases in GI absorption
  - Decrease in total body water (decreased plasma volume)
  - Decreased lean muscle and increased adipose tissue
  - Reduced first-pass effect in the liver and cardiac output
  - Decreased serum albumin
  - Decreased glomerular filtration and renal tubular secretion
  - Time to steady state is prolonged

Because of decrease in lean muscle mass and increase in fat (retains lipophilic drugs [fat-storing]), reduced first-pass metabolism, and decreased renal function, drugs may remain in the body longer and produce an additive effect.

ALERT: With the elderly, start doses low and titrate slowly. Drugs that result in postural hypotension, confusion, or sedation should be used cautiously or not at all.

- **Poor Drug Choices for the Elderly** – Drugs that cause postural hypotension or anticholinergic side effects (sedation).
  - *TCAs* – anticholinergic (confusion, constipation, visual blurring); cardiac (conduction delay; tachycardia); alpha-1 adrenergic (orthostatic hypotension [falls])
  - *Benzodiazepines* – longer the half-life; greater the risk of falls. Choose a shorter half-life. Lorazepam ($T^1/_2$ 12–15 h) is a better choice than diazepam ($T^1/_2$ 20–70 h; metabolites up to 200 h).
  - *Lithium* – use cautiously in elderly, especially if debilitated.
  - Consider age, weight, mental state, and medical disorders and compare with side-effect profile in selecting medications.

MAOI Diet (Tyramine) Restrictions

Foods: Must Avoid Completely

- Aged red wines (cabernet sauvignon/merlot/chianti)
- Aged (smoked, aged, pickled, fermented, marinated, and processed) meats (pepperoni/bologna/salami, pickled herring, liver, frankfurters, bacon, ham)
- Aged/mature cheeses (blue/cheddar/provolone/brie/romano/parmesan/Swiss)
- Overripe fruits and vegetables (overripe bananas/sauerkraut/all overripe fruit)
- Beans (fava, Italian, Chinese pea pod, fermented bean curd, soya sauce, tofu, Miso soup)
- Condiments (bouillon cubes/meat tenderizers/canned soups/gravy/sauces/ soy sauce)
- Soups (prepared/canned/frozen)
- Beverages (beer/ales/vermouth/whiskey/liqueurs/nonalcoholic wines and beers)

Foods: Use With Caution (Moderation)

- Avocados (not overripe)
- Raspberries (small amounts)
- Chocolate (small amount)
- Caffeine (2 – 8 oz. servings per day or less)
- Dairy products (limit to buttermilk, yogurt, and sour cream [small amounts]); cream cheese, cottage cheese, milk OK if fresh

Medications: Must Avoid

- Stimulants
- Decongestants
- OTC medications (check with PCP/pharmacist)
- Opioids
- Meperidine
- Ephedrine/epinephrine
- Methyldopa
- Herbal remedies

Any questions about foods, OTC medications, herbals, medications (newly prescribed) should be discussed with the psychiatrist, pharmacist, or advanced practice nurse because of serious nature of any food-drug, drug-drug combinations.

Neuroleptic Malignant Syndrome (NMS)

A serious and potentially fatal syndrome caused by antipsychotics and other drugs that block dopamine receptors. Important not to allow client to become *dehydrated* (predisposing factor). More common in warm climates, in summer. Possible genetic predisposition.

Signs and Symptoms

- Fever: 103°–105° F or greater
- Blood pressure lability (hypertension or hypotension)
- Tachycardia (>130 bpm)
- Tachypnea (>25 rpm)
- Agitation (respiratory distress, tachycardia)
- Diaphoresis, pallor
- Muscle rigidity (arm/abdomen like a board)
- Change in mental status (stupor to coma)
- Stop antipsychotic immediately.

ALERT: NMS is a medical emergency (10% mortality rate); hospitalization needed. Lab test: creatinine kinase (CK) to determine injury to the muscle. Drugs used to treat NMS include: bromocriptine, dantroline, levodopa, lorazepam.

Serotonin Syndrome

Can occur if client is taking one or more serotonergic drugs (e.g., SSRIs; also St. John's wort), especially higher doses. Do not combine SSRIs/SNRIs/clomipramine with MAOI; also tryptophan, dextromethorphan combined with MAOI can produce this syndrome.

If stopping fluoxetine (long half-life) to start an MAOI – must allow a 5-week washout period. At least 2 weeks for other SSRIs before starting an MAOI. Discontinue MAOI for 2 weeks before starting another antidepressant or other interacting drug.

Signs and Symptoms

- Change in mental status, agitation, confusion, restlessness, flushing
- Diaphoresis, diarrhea, lethargy
- Myoclonus (muscle twitching or jerks), tremors

If serotonergic medication is not discontinued, progresses to:

- Worsening myoclonus, hypertension, rigor
- Acidosis, respiratory failure, rhabdomyolysis

ALERT: Must discontinue serotonergic drug immediately. Emergency medical treatment and hospitalization needed to treat myoclonus, hypertension, and other symptoms.

Note: Refer to *Physicians' Desk Reference* or product insert for complete drug information (dosages, warnings, indications, adverse effects, interactions, etc.) needed to make appropriate choices in the treatment of clients. Although every effort has been made to provide key information about medications and classes of drugs, such information is not and cannot be all-inclusive in a reference of this nature. Professional judgment, training, supervision, relevant references, and current drug information is critical to the appropriate selection, evaluation, monitoring, and management of clients and their medications.

Labs/Plasma Levels

Therapeutic Plasma Levels — Mood Stabilizers

- Lithium: 1.0–1.5 mEq/L (acute mania)
  0.6–1.2 mEq/L (maintenance)
  Toxic: >2.0 mEq/L
- Carbamazepine: 4–12 μg/mL
  Toxic >15 μg/mL
- Valproic acid: 50–100 μg/mL

Note: Lithium blood level should be drawn in the morning about 12 hours after last oral dose and before first morning dose.

Plasma Level/Lab Test Monitoring

- **Lithium** – Initially check serum level every 1–2 wk (for at least 2 mo), then every 3–6 mo; renal function every 6–12 mo; TFTs every year.
- **Carbamazepine** – Serum levels every 1–2 wk (at least for 2 mo); CBC and LFTs every mo, then CBCs/LFTs every 6–12 mo; serum levels every 3–6 mo as appropriate.
- **Valproic acid** – Serum level checks every 1–2 wk; CBC/LFTs every mo; serum level every 3–6 mo; CBC/LFT every 6–12 mo.

Disorders and Labs/Tests

- Labs and tests should be performed on all clients before arriving at a diagnosis to rule out a physical cause that may mimic a psychological disorder and before starting treatments. Tests should be repeated as appropriate after diagnosis to monitor treatments/reevaluate.

Disorder	Labs/Tests
Anxiety	Physical exam, psych eval, mental status exam, TFTs (hyperthyroidism), CBC, general chemistry, toxicology screens (substance abuse); anxiety inventories/rating scales

Continued

Disorder	Labs/Tests
Dementia	Physical exam, psych eval, mental status exam, Mini-Mental State Exam, TFTs, LFTs, CBC, sed rate, general chemistry, toxicology screens (substance abuse), B_{12}, folate, UA, HIV, FTA-ABS (syphilis), depression inventories/rating scales (Geriatric Rating Scale), CT/MRI, Structural MRI (Vermuri 2010), CSF biomarkers (Andersson 2011)
Depression	Physical exam, psych eval, mental status exam, Mini-Mental State Exam (R/O dementia), TFTs (hypothyroidism), LFTs, CBC, general chemistry, toxicology screens (substance abuse); depression inventories/rating scales (R/O pseudodementia), CT/MRI
Mania	Physical exam, psych eval, mental status exam, Young Mania Rating Scale (bipolar I), Mood Disorder Questionnaire (see Assessment Tab), TFTs (hyperthyroidism), LFTs, toxicology screens (substance abuse), CBC, UA, ECG (>40 y), serum levels (VA, CBZ, Li), BMI, general chemistry/metabolic panel, pregnancy test, CT/MRI
Postpartum depression	Physical exam, psych eval (history of previous depression/psychosis), mental status exam, TFTs, CBC, general chemistry, Edinburgh Postnatal Depression Scale, monitor/screen during postpartal period (fathers also)
Schizophrenia	Physical exam, psych eval, mental status exam, TFTs (hyperthyroidism), LFTs, toxicology screens (substance abuse), CBC, UA, serum glucose, BMI, general chemistry/metabolic panel, VeriPsych biomarker blood test (VeriPsych 2010), pregnancy test, CT/MRI; Positive and Negative Syndrome Scale, AIMs

Clozaril Protocol – Clozaril Patient Management System

Indications for use: Patients with a diagnosis of schizophrenia, unresponsive or intolerant to *three* different neuroleptics from at least *two* different therapeutic groups, when given adequate doses for adequate duration.

- System for monitoring WBCs of patients on clozapine. Important because of *possible (life-threatening) agranulocytosis and leukopenia.*
- Need to monitor WBCs, absolute neutrophil count (ANC), and differential before initiating therapy and after.
- WBC and ANC weekly first 6 mo, then bi-weekly, then weekly for 1 month after discontinuation.

Continued

- Only available in 1-wk supply (requires WBCs, patient monitoring, and controlled distribution through pharmacies).
- If WBC <3000 mm^3 or granulocyte count <1500 mm^3 – withhold clozapine (monitor for signs & symptoms of infection).
- Monthly monitoring approved under certain situations (FDA approval 2005).
- Patients must be registered with the Clozaril National Registry (see www.clozaril.com).

General Chemistry

NOTE: Reference ranges vary according to brand of laboratory assay materials used. Check normal reference ranges from your facility's laboratory when evaluating results.

Lab	Conventional	SI Units
Albumin	3.5–5.0 g/100 mL	35–50 g/L
Aldolase	1.3–8.2 U/L	22–137 nmol sec^{-1}/L
Alkaline phosphatase	42–136 U/L	217–650 nmol · sec^{-1}/ L, up to 1.26 µmol/L
Ammonia	15–45 µg/dL	11–35 µmol/L
Amylase	4–25 units/mL	4–25 arb. unit
Anion gap	8–16 mEq/L	8–16 mmol/L
AST, SGOT	Male: 15–40 U/L Female: 13–35 U/L	15–40 U/L 13–35 U/L
Bilirubin, direct	Up to 0.4 mg/100 mL	Up to 7 µmol/L
Bilirubin, total	Up to 1.0 mg/100 mL	Up to 17 µmol/L
BUN	8–25 mg/100 mL	2.9–8.9 mmol/L
Ca^+ (calcium)	8.5–10.5 mg/100 mL	2.1–2.6 mmol/L
Calcitonin	Male: <19 pg/mL Female: <14 pg/mL	<19 ng/L <14 ng/L
Carbon dioxide (CO_2)	24–30 mEq/L	24–30 mmol/L
Chloride (Cl^-)	100–106 mEq/L	100–106 mmol/L
Cholesterol	<200 mg/dL	<5.18 mmol/L
Cortisol	(AM) 5–25 µg/100 mL (PM) <10 µg/100 mL	0.14–0.69 µmol/L 0–0.28 µmol/L
Creatine	Male: 0.2–0.5 mg/dL Female: 0.3–0.9 mg/dL	15–40 µmol/L 25–70 µmol/L

Continued

Lab	Conventional	SI Units
Creatine kinase (CK)	Male: 50–204 U/L Female: 36–160 U/L	50–204 U/L 36–160 U/L
Creatinine	0.6–1.5 mg/100 mL	53–133 µmol/L
Ferritin	10–410 ng/dL	10–410 µg/dL
Folate	2.0–9.0 ng/mL	4.5–0.4 nmol/L
Glucose	70–110 mg/100 mL	3.9–5.6 mmol/L
Ionized calcium	4.25–5.25 mg/dL	1.1–1.3 mmol/L
Iron (Fe)	50–150 µg/100 mL	9.0–26.9 µmol/L
Iron binding capacity (IBC)	250–410 µg/100 mL	44.8–73.4 µmol/L
K^+ (potassium)	3.5–5.0 mEq/L	3.5–5.0 mmol/L
Lactic acid	0.6–1.8 mEq/L	0.6–1.8 mmol/L
LDH (lactic dehydrogenase)	45–90 U/L	750–1500 nmol · sec^{-1}/L
Lipase	2 units/mL or less	Up to 2 arb. unit
Magnesium	1.5–2.0 mEq/L	0.8–1.3 mmol/L
Mg^{++} (magnesium)	1.5–2.0 mEq/L	0.8–1.3 mmol/L
Na^+ (sodium)	135–145 mEq/L	135–145 mmol/L
Osmolality	280–296 mOsm/kg water	280–296 mmol/kg
Phosphorus	3.0–4.5 mg/100 mL	1.0–1.5 mmol/L
Potassium (K^+)	3.5–5.0 mEq/L	3.5–5.0 mmol/L
Prealbumin	18–32 mg/dL	180–320 mg/L
Protein, total	6.0–8.4 g/100 mL	60–84 g/L
PSA	<4.0 ng/mL	<4 µg/L
Pyruvate	0–0.11 mEq/L	0–0.11 mmol/L
Sodium (Na^+)	135–145 mEq/L	135–145 mmol/L
T3	75–195 ng/100 mL	1.16–3.00 nmol/L
T4, free	Male: 0.8–1.8 ng/dL Female: 0.8–1.8 ng/dL	10–23 pmol/L 10–23 pmol/L
T4, total	4–12 µg/100 mL	52–154 nmol/L
Thyroglobulin	3–42 µ/mL	3–42 µg/L
Triglycerides	40–150 mg/100 mL	0.4–1.5 g/L
TSH	0.5–5.0 µU/mL	0.5–5.0 arb. unit
Urea nitrogen	8–25 mg/100 mL	2.9–8.9 mmol/L
Uric acid	3.0–7.0 mg/100 mL	0.18–0.42 mmol/L

Hematology

Lab	Conventional	SI Units
Blood volume	8.5%–9.0% of body weight in kg	80–85 mL/kg
Red Blood Cell **(RBC)**	Male: 4.6–6.2 million/mm^3 Female: 4.2–5.9 million/mm^3	4.6–6.2 × 10^{12}/L 4.2–5.9 × 10^{12}/L
Hemoglobin **(Hgb)**	Male: 13–18 g/100 mL Female: 12–16 g/100 mL	Male: 8.1–11.2 mmol/L Female: 7.4–9.9 mmol/L
Hematocrit **(Hct)**	Male: 45%–52% Female: 37%–48%	Male: 0.45–0.52 Female: 0.37–0.48
Leukocytes **(WBC)**	4,300–10,800/mm^3	4.3–10.8 × 10^9/L
• Bands	0–5%	0.03–0.08 × 10^9/L
• Basophils	0–1%	0–0.01 × 10^9/L
• Eosinophils	1%–4%	0.01–0.04 × 10^9/L
• Lymphocytes	25%–40%	0.25–0.40 × 10^9/L
• *B-Lymphocytes*	10%–20%	0.10–0.20 × 10^9/L
• *T-Lymphocytes*	60%–80%	0.60–0.80 × 10^9/L
• Monocytes	2%–8%	0.02–0.08 × 10^9/L
• Neutrophils	54%–75%	0.54–0.75 × 10^9/L
Platelets	150,000–350,000/mm^3	150–350 × 10^9/L
Erythrocyte Sedimentation Rate (ESR)	Male: 1–13 mm/hr Female: 1–20 mm/hr	Male: 1–13 mm/hr Female: 1–20 mm/hr

Thyroid Panel

T_3 Total	75–195 ng/100 mL	1.16–3.00 nmol/L
T_3 Uptake (RT_3U)	25%–35%	0.25–0.35
T_3 Uptake Ratio	0.1–1.35	0.1–0.35
T_4 Total	4–12 μg/100 mL	52–154 nmol/L
T_4 Free	0.9–2.3 ng/dL	10–30 nm/L
TSH	0.5–5.0 μU/mL	0.5–5.0 arb. Unit

Renal/Kidney

Lab	Conventional	SI Units
BUN	6–23 mg/dL	2.5–7.5 mmol/L
Creatinine	15–25 mg/kg of body weight/day	0.13–0.22 mmol kg^{-1}/day
Uric acid	Male: 4.0–9.0 mg/dL Female: 3.0–6.5 mg/dL	238–535 µmol/L 178–387 µmol/L

Urinalysis (UA)

Color	Yellow-straw
Specific Gravity	1.005–1.030
pH	5.0–8.0
Glucose	Negative
Sodium	10–40 mEq/L
Potassium	<8 mEq/L
Chloride	<8 mEq/L
Protein	Negative-trace
Osmolality	500–800 mOsm/L

Psychotropic Drugs A – Z

The following drugs are listed alphabetically within this tab by generic name (example trade name in parentheses):

* Latest drugs approved/released into the marketplace.

NOTE: See QR barcode on the inside front cover of this book to immediately access 78 complete psychotropic drug monographs (using a downloaded app on your smartphone) or access online at DavisPlus at: http://davisplus.fadavis.com.

Psychotropic Drugs A – Z (Alphabetical Listing)

Psychotropic Drug Tables that follow include each drug's half life (T½), protein binding, pregnancy categories, Canadian drug trade names *(in italics)*, dose ranges and adult doses, most common side effects (CSE), geriatric and dose considerations, and LIFE-THREATENING (ALL CAPS) side effects, listed alphabetically by generic name. *(See Alert at end of tab as well as FDA Warnings.)*

Generic (Trade)	Dose Range/ Adult Daily Dose	Use/Common Side Effects (CSE)	Geriatric & Dose Considerations	Classification Assessment Cautions
Alprazolam (Xanax, Xanax XR, *Apo-Alpraz, Novo-Alprazol, Nu-Alpraz*) Intermediate T½ = 12–15 h Pregnancy category D	0.25–0.5 mg po 2–3 times daily (anxiety); *panic*: 0.5 mg 3 times daily; not to exceed 10 mg/d; *XR:* 0.5–1 mg once daily in AM; usual range 3–6 mg/d	*Use:* Anxiety, panic; *unlabeled:* PMS *CSE:* Dizziness, drowsiness, lethargy; sometimes confusion, hangover, paradoxical excitation, constipation, diarrhea, nausea, vomiting	↓ Dose required; begin 0.25 mg 2–3 times/d; assess CNS and risk for falls; Elderly have ↑ sensitivity to benzodiazepines.	Antianxiety agent Monitor CBC, liver, renal function in long-term therapy; avoid grapefruit juice; risk for psychological/physical dependence; seizures on abrupt discontinuation. Interacts with alcohol, antidepressants, antihistamines, other benzos and opioids.

Continued

Psychotropic Drugs A – Z (Alphabetical Listing)—cont'd

Generic (Trade)	Dose Range/ Adult Daily Dose	Use/Common Side Effects (CSE)	Geriatric & Dose Considerations	Classification **Assessment** **Cautions**
Amitriptyline (Elavil, *Apo-Amitriptyline*) T½ = 10–50 h Protein binding = >95% Pregnancy category C	Range: 50–300 mg/d; dosage: 75 mg/d po in divided doses up to 150 mg/d or 50–100 mg hs; increase by 25–50 mg to 150 mg (in hospital: start 100 mg/d up to 300 mg)	*Use:* Depression; *unlabeled:* chronic pain *CSE:* Blurred vision, dry eyes, dry mouth, sedation, hypotension, constipation, ARRHYTHMIAS	Use caution: Orthostatic hypotension, sedation, confusion (falls); CV disease; titrate slowly	Antidepressant [TCA] Hx CV disease or high doses: *Monitor* ECG prior to and through Rx

Continued

Psychotropic Drugs A – Z (Alphabetical Listing)—cont'd

Generic (Trade)	Dose Range/ Adult Daily Dose	Use/Common Side Effects (CSE)	Geriatric & Dose Considerations	Classification Assessment Cautions
Aripiprazole (Abilify, Abilify Discmelt, Abilify Oral Solution and Injection) T½ = 75 h; dehydroaripiprazole = 94 h Protein binding = >99% T½ = 2–3 h Pregnancy category C	*Schizophrenia:* 10–15 mg/d po (up to 30 mg/d); ↑ only after 2 wk at a given dose. *Bipolar I (acute manic/mixed):* start 15 mg/d (up to 30 mg/d) *Agitation* (schizophrenia or bipolar): *IM* – 9.75 mg; range 5.25–15 mg See Prescribing info for adjunct Rx	*Use:* Schizophrenia, acute bipolar mania (manic/mixed/ maintenance); *MDD:* augmentation of standard antidepressant therapy; Autistic irritability; IM: Agitation (bipolar/ schizophrenia) *CSE:* Nausea, anxiety, confusion, constipation, orthostatic hypotension, ↑ salivation, ecchymoses, NMS	Orthostatic hypotension; caution with CV disease; ↑ mortality in elderly with dementia-related psychosis	Antipsychotic [Atypical] *Contraindicated:* Lactation; caution with CV/cerebrovascular diseases; avoid dehydration; NEUROLEPTIC MALIGNANT SYNDROME *Monitor* BMI, FBS, and lipids

Continued

Psychotropic Drugs A – Z (Alphabetical Listing)—cont'd

Generic (Trade)	Dose Range/ Adult Daily Dose	Use/Common Side Effects (CSE)	Geriatric & Dose Considerations	Classification Assessment Cautions
Asenapine (Saphris) T½ = 24 h Protein binding = 95% Sublingual (SL) Pregnancy category C	*Schizophrenia* (*acute*): 5 mg SL twice daily; *maintenance*: start 5 mg SL twice daily X 1 wk, to 10 mg SL twice daily *Bipolar mania (monotherapy)*: start 10 mg SL twice daily to 5–10 mg SL twice daily; *adjunct to lithium/valproate*: 5 mg twice daily to 5–10 mg twice daily; maximum dose: 10 mg twice daily	*Use*: *Schizophrenia,* acute and maintenance; *Bipolar I,* acute mania and mixed episodes; and adjunctive therapy with lithium or valproate *CSE*: *schizophrenia:* akathisia, somnolence, oral hypoesthesia *Bipolar*: somnolence, dizziness, EPS other than akathisia, weight gain	Caution in elderly because of orthostatic hypotension, dizziness, or somnolence. Start at lowest dose. Only 1.1% of clinical trial patients were >65. *Warning:* ↑mortality in elderly with dementia-related psychosis	Antipsychotic [Atypical] *Caution*: coadministration w *fluvoxamine (strong CYP1A2 inhibitor) and paroxetine (CYP2D6 substrate and inhibitor);* No adjustment needed for renal impairment, do not use with severe hepatic impairment. Caution with alcohol, and other centrally acting drugs, and antihypertensive agents. *Assess*: Monitor for suicidality early on and throughout Rx. TD, NMS, DM, orthostatic hypotension, QT prolongation, seizures

Continued

Psychotropic Drugs A – Z (Alphabetical Listing)—cont'd

Generic (Trade)	Dose Range/ Adult Daily Dose	Use/Common Side Effects (CSE)	Geriatric & Dose Considerations	Classification Assessment Cautions
Benztropine (Cogentin, *Apo-Benztropine)* T½ = Unknown Pregnancy category C	*Parkinsonism:* 0.5–6 mg/d *EPS:* PO/IM/IV: 1–4 mg qd or bid or 1–2 mg po 2–3 times daily; *acute dystonia:* IM/IV: 1–2 mg; then 1–2 mg po bid	*Use:* Parkinson's, drug-induced EPS, and acute dystonia *CSE:* Blurred vision, dry mouth, dry eyes, constipation, urinary retention	Use cautiously; ↑ risk of adverse reactions	Antiparkinson agent *Contraindicated:* Narrow-angle glaucoma and TD; Assess parkinsonian/ EPS symptoms; bowel function (constipation)/ urinary retention *IM/IV:* Monitor pulse/ BP closely; advise slow position changes
Bupropion (Wellbutrin, Wellbutrin SR, Wellbutrin XL) Bupropion hydro-bromide (Aplenzin) [Once daily dosing] T½ = 14 h (metabolites possibly longer) Pregnancy category B	*IR:* 100 mg po bid; after 3 d ↑ to tid; wk 4 to 450 mg/d in divided doses, not to exceed 150 mg/dose *Aplenzin:* 348 mg/d once in AM; start 174 mg/d, ↑ after 4 d to *max:* 522 mg/d	*Use:* Depression; adult ADHD (SR only); ↑ female sexual desire *CSE:* Agitation, headache, dry mouth, nausea, vomiting, SEIZURES	Use cautiously; ↑ risk of drug accumulation	Antidepressant *Contraindicated:* Hx bulimia or anorexia; seizure disorder Seizure risk ↑ at doses >450 mg; **avoid alcohol**

Continued

Psychotropic Drugs A – Z (Alphabetical Listing)—cont'd

Generic (Trade)	Dose Range/ Adult Daily Dose	Use/Common Side Effects (CSE)	Geriatric & Dose Considerations	Classification Assessment Cautions
Buspirone (BuSpar) T½ = 2–3 h Protein binding = >95% Pregnancy category B	15–60 mg/d po	*Use:* Anxiety management; anxiety w depression *CSE:* Dizziness, drowsiness, blurred vision, palpitations, chest pain, nausea, rashes, myalgia, sweating	*Contraindicated:* Severe renal/ hepatic disease	Antianxiety agent *Contraindicated:* Severe renal/hepatic impairment; does not appear to cause dependence
Carbamazepine (Tegretol, Tegretol XR, Equetro, Epitol, *Apo-Carbamazepine, Tegretol CR*) T½ = single dose = 25–65 h; chronic dosing = 8–29 h Pregnancy category D	*Start:* 200 mg/d or 100 mg bid; increase weekly by 200 mg/d until therapeutic level/ mania improvement. *Equetro (Bipolar):* 400 mg/d divided doses, twice daily up to 1600 mg/d	*Use:* Bipolar I: Acute mania/mixed (Equetro); *CSE:* Ataxia, drowsiness, blurred vision. APLASTIC ANEMIA, AGRANULOCYTOSIS, THROMBOCYTOPENIA, STEVENS-JOHNSON SYNDROME (SJS)	Use cautiously; CV/hepatic disease; BPH and increased intraocular pressure	Anticonvulsant/ mood stabilizer *Caution:* Impaired liver/cardiac functions. Monitor CBC, platelets, reticulocytes. HLA-B* 1502 typing for those genetically at risk (Asians). Therpeutic Range (4–12 mg/mL). *Sx of SJS:* cough, FUO, mucosal lesions, rash; stop CBZ

Continued

Psychotropic Drugs A – Z (Alphabetical Listing)—cont'd

Generic (Trade)	Dose Range/ Adult Daily Dose	Use/Common Side Effects (CSE)	Geriatric & Dose Considerations	Classification Assessment Cautions
Chlordiazepoxide (Librium, Libritabs, *Apo-Chlordiazepoxide*; Librax [comb w clidinium], Limbitrol DS [comb w amitriptyline]) $T½$ = 5–30 h Pregnancy category D	*Anxiety:* 5–25 mg po 3–4 × daily *Alcohol withdrawal:* IM: 50–100 mg; may repeat in 3–4 h or po 50–100 mg; repeat until agitation ↓ (to 400 mg/d)	*Use:* Adjunct anxiety management; alcohol withdrawal *CSE:* Dizziness, drowsiness, pain at IM site	May cause prolonged sedation in the elderly and is associated with ↑ risk of falls. Must reduce dose or consider short-acting benzodiazepine.	Antianxiety agent [benzo] *Contraindicated:* Narrow-angle glaucoma, porphyria; caution with hepatic/renal impairment and history of suicide attempt/substance abuse
Chlorpromazine (Thorazine, Thor-Prom, *Chlorpromanyl, Largactil, Novo-Chlorpromazine*) $T½$ = initial 2 h; end 30 h Protein binding = ≥ 90% Pregnancy category unknown	*Range:* 40–800 mg/d po *Psychoses:* 10–25 mg po 2–4 times/d; may ↑ q 3–4 d up to 1 g/d; IM: Start 25–50 mg IM to max. 400 mg q 3–12 h (max. 1 g/d)	*Use:* Psychosis; combativeness CSE: Hypotension (esp IM), dry eyes, sedation, blurred vision, constipation, dry mouth, photosensitivity, NMS, AGRANULOCYTOSIS	*Caution:* Sedating; decrease initial dose. *Caution*: BPH	Antipsychotic [Conventional] *Contraindicated:* Glaucoma, bone marrow depression, severe liver/ CV disease. *Monitor* BP, pulse, and respirations, CBCs, LFTs, and eye exams; EPS, akathisia, NMS

Continued

Psychotropic Drugs A – Z (Alphabetical Listing)—cont'd

Generic (Trade)	Dose Range/ Adult Daily Dose	Use/Common Side Effects (CSE)	Geriatric & Dose Considerations	Classification Assessment Cautions
Citalopram (Celexa) T½ = 35 h Pregnancy category C	*Range:* 20–60 mg/d po Start 20 mg po daily, increased weekly, if needed, by 20 mg/d up to 60 mg/d (usual dose: 40 mg/d)	*Use:* Depression *CSE:* Apathy, confusion, drowsiness, insomnia, abdominal pain, anorexia, diarrhea, dyspepsia, nausea, sweating, tremor	20 mg po once daily; may increase to 40 mg/d only in those not responding. Lower doses with hepatic/renal impairment.	Antidepressant [SSRI] *Contraindicated:* Use within 14 days of MAOI; *Caution:* hx of mania or seizures; serotonin syndrome with SAMe or St. John's wort; monitor for mood changes and assess for suicide
Clomipramine (Anafranil, *Apo-Clomipramine*) T½ = 20–30 h Pregnancy category C	*Range:* 25–250 mg/d po Start 25 mg/d po; gradually increase to 100 mg/d (up to 250 mg/d)	*Use:* OCD *CSE:* Dizziness, drowsiness, increased appetite, weight gain, constipation, nausea	Use with caution in elderly (sedation, orthostatic hypotension; CV disease; BPH)	Antidepressant [TCA] *Caution:* CV disease including conduction abnormalities, hx: seizures, bipolar, hypotensive disorders; avoid alcohol; *fatal with MAOIs.*

Continued

Psychotropic Drugs A – Z (Alphabetical Listing)—cont'd

Generic (Trade)	Dose Range/ Adult Daily Dose	Use/Common Side Effects (CSE)	Geriatric & Dose Considerations	Classification **Assessment** **Cautions**
Clonazepam (Klonopin, *Rivotril, Syn-Clonazepam*) T½ = 18–50 h Schedule IV Pregnancy category D	*Range:* 1.5–4 mg/d po (panic/anxiety); as high as 6 mg/d; up to 20 mg/d for seizures	*Use:* Panic disorder, seizure disorders; restless leg syndrome *CSE:* Behavioral changes, drowsiness, ataxia	*Caution:* Drowsiness; *Contraindicated:* Liver disease	Antianxiety agent [benzo] *Contraindicated:* Severe liver disease; *assess* for drowsiness: dose-related. *Monitor:* CBC/LFTs with prolonged therapy
Clozapine (Clozaril, FazaClo) T½ = 8–12 h Protein binding = 95% [FazaClo—orally disintegrating tablets] Pregnancy category B	*Range:* 300–900 mg/d po Start 25 mg po 1–2 × daily; ↑ 25–50 mg/d over 2 wk up to 300–450 mg/d (not to exceed 900 mg/d) FazaClo: start 12.5 mg 1–2 × daily; no water needed	*Use:* Refractive schizophrenia (unresponsive to other treatments) *CSE:* Dizziness, sedation, hypotension, tachycardia, constipation, NMS, SEIZURES, AGRANULOCYTOSIS, LEUKOPENIA, MYOCARDITIS (D/C clozapine)	Use cautiously with CV/hepatic/ renal disease; sedating; ↑ mortality in elderly with dementia-related psychosis	Antipsychotic [Atypical] *Must follow Clozaril protocol: Monitor* BP/pulse; CBC (WBC/diff <3000/mm³—withhold clozapine). (See Clozaril Protocol in Drug-Lab Tab) *Monitor* for signs of myocarditis akathisia, EPS, and NMS; also BMI, FBS, and lipids. (For FazaClo Protocol, see www.Fazaclo.com)

Continued

Psychotropic Drugs A – Z (Alphabetical Listing)—cont'd

Generic (Trade)	Dose Range/ Adult Daily Dose	Use/Common Side Effects (CSE)	Geriatric & Dose Considerations	Classification **Assessment Cautions**
Desipramine (Norpramin, *Pertofrane*) T½ = 12–27 h Protein binding = 90%–92% Pregnancy category C	*Range:* 25–300 mg/d 100–200 mg/d po single or divided doses (up to 300 mg/d)	*Use:* Depression; *unlabeled:* chronic pain *CSE:* Blurred vision, dry eyes, dry mouth, sedation, hypotension, constipation ARRHYTHMIAS	*Reduce dosage:* 25–50 mg/d po (in divided doses (up to 150 mg/d); sedation. *Caution* with CV disease, BPH; monitor BP & pulse	Antidepressant [TCA] *Contraindicated:* Narrow-angle glaucoma. *Monitor* BP/pulse; ECG prior to and through Rx if hx of CV disease or high doses

Continued

Psychotropic Drugs A – Z (Alphabetical Listing)—cont'd

Generic (Trade)	Dose Range/ Adult Daily Dose	Use/Common Side Effects (CSE)	Geriatric & Dose Considerations	Classification Assessment Cautions
Desvenlafaxine (Pristiq) T½ = 11 h Pregnancy category C	*Adults:* 50 mg po once daily; in clinical studies (50–400 mg/d) there did not seem to be additional benefit above 50 mg/d. The recommended dose with moderate renal impairment (24-hr CrCl = 30–50 mL/min) is 50 mg/d; with severe renal impairment (24-hr CrCl < 30 mL/min) or end-stage renal disease (ESRD) 50 mg every other day. *Extended release formulation* (once-daily dosing) should not be chewed or crushed	*Use:* Major depressive disorder in adults only *CSE*: Anxiety, dizziness, headache, abnormal dreams, insomnia, nervousness, weakness, mydriasis, rhinitis, visual disturbances, anorexia, constipation, diarrhea, dry mouth, dyspepsia, nausea, vomiting, weight loss, sexual dysfunction, ecchymoses, paresthesias, chills	*Caution* in elderly with CV disease, hypertension, liver or renal impairment, and hx of increased intraocular pressure, or narrow-angle glaucoma. *Monitor* for suicidality and see dosing for renal impairment.	Antidepressant [SNRI] Concurrent MAOI therapy is contraindicated. Use with alcohol, CNS depressants not recommended. Beware of multiple drug-drug interactions; no adjustment needed for mild/ moderate hepatic/ renal impairment (hepatic impairment: max dose 100 mg/d). *Caution* with preexisting hypertension; hypertension dose-related. Assess: monitor for suicidality early on and throughout Rx. Also BP before/ after Rx (↓ dose or D/C). Taper slowly to D/C.

Continued

Psychotropic Drugs A – Z (Alphabetical Listing)—cont'd

Generic (Trade)	Dose Range/ Adult Daily Dose	Use/Common Side Effects (CSE)	Geriatric & Dose Considerations	Classification Assessment Cautions
Diazepam (Valium, *Apo-Diazepam, Vivol*) $T_{1/2}$ = 20–50 h (up to 100 h for metabolites) Schedule IV Pregnancy category D	*Range:* 4–40 mg/d *Anxiety: po*: 2–10 mg 2–4 × daily; *IM/IV*: 2–10 mg q 4 h prn. *Alcohol WD: po:* 10 mg 3–4 × first 24 h; then 5 mg 3–4 × daily; *IM/IV*: 10 mg, then 5–10 mg in 3–4 h as needed	*Use:* Anxiety adjunct; alcohol withdrawal *CSE:* Dizziness, drowsiness, lethargy	Dosage reduction required; *caution:* hepatic/renal disease; *assess:* risk for falls; prolonged sedation in the elderly	Antianxiety agent [benzo] *Monitor:* BP/pulse/ respirations; CBC, LFTs; renal tests periodically with prolonged therapy; *Monitor* for dependence. *Alcoholics:* ETOH withdrawal–*assess for:* tremors, delirium, agitation, hallucinations

Continued

Psychotropic Drugs A – Z (Alphabetical Listing)—cont'd

Generic (Trade)	Dose Range/ Adult Daily Dose	Use/Common Side Effects (CSE)	Geriatric & Dose Considerations	Classification **Assessment** **Cautions**
Divalproex sodium (Depakote, Depakote ER, *Epival*) [Valproate] T½ = 5–20 h Pregnancy category D	*Range:* 500–1500 mg/d po [up to 4000 mg/d] *Initially:* 750 mg/d in divided doses, titrated to clinical effect/plasma levels; *ER:* Single dose at bedtime	*Use:* Bipolar, acute mania & prophylaxis *CSE:* Nausea, vomiting, indigestion, HEPATOTOXICITY, PANCREATITIS	*Caution* with renal impairment, organic brain disease, assess for excessive somnolence	Anticonvulsant/ mood stabilizer *Contraindicated:* Hepatic impairment; *Monitor* LFTs, serum ammonia before and throughout Rx Hyperammonemia: D/C VA. *Caution:* Renal/ bleeding disorders; bone marrow depression; *teratogenicity;* need VA levels (50–100 μg/mL)

Continued

Psychotropic Drugs A – Z (Alphabetical Listing)—cont'd

Generic (Trade)	Dose Range/ Adult Daily Dose	Use/Common Side Effects (CSE)	Geriatric & Dose Considerations	Classification Assessment Cautions
Doxepin (Sinequan, Zonalon, *Triadapin*) $T\frac{1}{2}$ = 8–25 h Pregnancy category C	*Range:* 25–300 mg/d po 25 mg po 3 × daily, up to 150 mg (inpatient up to 300 mg/d)	*Use:* Depression/ anxiety *CSE:* Blurred vision, dry eyes, dry mouth, sedation, hypotension, constipation, ARRHYTHMIAS	*Dose reduction:* 25–50 mg/d po initially, increase as needed; *Caution* with preexisting CV disease, BPH; *assess* for falls and anticholinergic effects	Antidepressant [TCA] *Monitor* blood pressure and pulse; ECGs with hx of CV disease; WBC w diff, LFTs, and serum glucose periodically
Duloxetine (Cymbalta) $T\frac{1}{2}$ = 12 h Protein binding = >90% Pregnancy category C	*Range:* 40–60 mg/d; 20–30 mg po twice daily	*Use:* Major depressive disorder *CSE:* fatigue, drowsiness, insomnia, ↓ appetite, constipation, dry mouth, nausea, dysuria, ↑ sweating, SEIZURES	Use with *caution*; increase slowly	Antidepressant [SNRI] *Contraindicated:* Concurrent MAOIs, hepatic impairment/ETOH use; with renal impairment: start with lower dose. *Monitor* BP (↑ BP dose-related) & LFTs; *monitor* for suicidality

Continued

Psychotropic Drugs A – Z (Alphabetical Listing)—cont'd

Generic (Trade)	Dose Range/ Adult Daily Dose	Use/Common Side Effects (CSE)	Geriatric & Dose Considerations	Classification Assessment Cautions
Escitalopram (Lexapro) T½ = increased in hepatic impairment Pregnancy category C	*Range:* 10–20 mg/d; 10 mg po once daily, may increase to 20 mg/d after 1 wk	*Use:* Depression, generalized anxiety disorder *CSE:* Insomnia, diarrhea, nausea, sexual dysfunction	↓ dose in elderly; caution with hepatic/renal impairment (10 mg po once daily); T½ increased in the elderly	Antidepressant [SSRI] *Contraindicated:* Concurrent MAOIs or citalopram *Caution:* hx mania/ seizures or risk for suicide; *monitor* for suicidality
Eszopiclone (Lunesta) T½ = 6 h Protein binding = weakly bound Schedule IV Pregnancy category C	*Range:* 1–3 mg po Start at 2 mg po hs, may ↑ to 3 mg if needed	*Use:* Insomnia: Sleep latency/maintenance *CSE:* Anxiety, confusion, depression, headache, migraine, dizziness, hallucinations	Elderly should start with 1 mg po dose and take *immediately before* bedtime; should not exceed 2 mg/hs	Sedative/hypnotic *Severe hepatic impairment:* Start 1 mg. *Caution:* Concomitant illness, drug/ETOH abuse, psychiatric illness, abrupt withdrawal (see FDA warning, end of tab)

Continued

Psychotropic Drugs A – Z (Alphabetical Listing)—cont'd

Generic (Trade)	Dose Range/ Adult Daily Dose	Use/Common Side Effects (CSE)	Geriatric & Dose Considerations	Classification Assessment Cautions
Fluoxetine (Prozac, Prozac Weekly, Serafem [PMDD]) $T\frac{1}{2}$ = 1–3 d (norfluoxetine: 5–7 d) Protein binding = 94.5% Pregnancy category C	*Range:* 20–80 mg po *Depression/OCD:* Start 20 mg/d po, may ↑ weekly up to 80 mg; *Panic disorder:* Start 10 mg/d po up to 60 mg/d; *Prozac Weekly:* 90 mg/wk *Serafem:* start 20 mg/d up to 60 mg/d or start 14 days before menstruation	*Use:* Depression (also geriatric), OCD, bulimia nervosa, panic disorder *CSE:* Anxiety, drowsiness, headache, insomnia, nervousness, diarrhea, sexual dysfunction, ↑ sweating, pruritus, tremor	*Starting dose:* 10 mg/d (not to exceed 60 mg); *Caution* with hepatic/renal impairment and with multiple medications (long $T\frac{1}{2}$); Elderly at risk for excessive CNS stimulation, sleep disturbances, and agitation.	Antidepressant [SSRI] Serious fatal reactions with MAOIs, long washout needed. *Caution:* Hepatic/renal/ pregnancy/seizures. *Peds/Adol (18–24 y):* May increase risk of suicidal thinking and behavior; *must closely monitor*

Continued

Psychotropic Drugs A – Z (Alphabetical Listing)—cont'd

Generic (Trade)	Dose Range/ Adult Daily Dose	Use/Common Side Effects (CSE)	Geriatric & Dose Considerations	Classification Assessment Cautions
Fluphenazine hydrochloride (Prolixin, *Apo-Fluphenazine*) T½ = 4.7–15.3 h Fluphenazine decanoate (Prolixin Decanoate, *Modecate)* T½ = 6.8–9.6 d *Fluphenazine Enanthate* T½ = 3.7 d Protein binding ≥ 90% Pregnancy category C	*Range:* 1–40 mg/d *Fluphenazine HCl:* Start: 2.5–10 mg/d po (divided dose q 6–8 h); maintenance: 1–5 mg/d; *IM*: 1.25–2.5 mg q 6–8 h *Decanoate:* Start 12.5–25 mg IM/SC q 1–4 wk (may ↑ to 100 mg/dose)	*Use:* Psychotic disorders, schizophrenia, chronic schizophrenia *CSE:* EPS, photosensitivity, sedation, tardive dyskinesia, AGRANULOCYTOSIS	Use lower doses: *Fluphenazine HCl:* Start with 1–2.5 mg/d po; caution with BPH, respiratory disease; *Contraindicated:* severe liver/ CV disease; ↑ mortality in elderly with dementia-related psychosis	Antipsychotic [Conventional] *Contraindicated:* Severe liver/CV disease, use with pimozide, glaucoma, bone marrow depression *Monitor* BP, pulse, respiration, ECG changes, EPS, akathisia, TD, NMS (report immediately). Periodic CBCs, LFTs, eye exams

Continued

Psychotropic Drugs A – Z (Alphabetical Listing)—cont'd

Generic (Trade)	Dose Range/ Adult Daily Dose	Use/Common Side Effects (CSE)	Geriatric & Dose Considerations	Classification Assessment Cautions
Flurazepam (Dalmane, *Apo-Flurazepam, Somnol*) $T_{1/2}$ = 2.3 h (active metabolite may be 30–200 h) Protein binding = 97% Schedule IV Pregnancy category X	*Range:* 15–30 mg *Usual dose:* 15–30 mg po hs	*Use:* Short-term insomnia management (<4 wk) *CSE:* Drowsiness, confusion, dizziness, paradoxical excitation, blurred vision, constipation	Initial dose ↓: 15 mg po initially hs; hepatic disease; warn patient and family about ↑ risk for falls and requires assessment for falls and fall prevention	Sedative/hypnotic [benzo] *Contraindicated:* CNS depression, narrow-angle glaucoma, pregnancy, lactation. *Caution:* Hepatic disease, hx suicide attempts, avoid alcohol (see FDA warning, end of tab)
Fluvoxamine (Luvox) $T_{1/2}$ = 13.6–15.6 h Pregnancy category C	*Range:* 50–300 mg/d *Start:* 50 mg/d po hs, ↑ 50 mg q 4–7 d (divide equally, if dose >100 mg) (do not exceed 300 mg/d)	*Use:* OCD. *Off label:* depression, GAD, PTSD. *CSE:* Headache, dizziness, drowsiness, nervousness, insomnia, nausea, diarrhea, constipation	Reduce dose, titrate slowly; caution with impaired hepatic function	Antidepressant [SSRI] Serious fatal reactions with MAOIs. *Peds/Adol (18–24 y):* Weigh risk vs benefit. *Monitor* closely for suicidality

Continued

Psychotropic Drugs A – Z (Alphabetical Listing)—cont'd

Generic (Trade)	Dose Range/ Adult Daily Dose	Use/Common Side Effects (CSE)	Geriatric & Dose Considerations	Classification Assessment Cautions
Gabapentin (Neurontin, Gabarone) T½ = 5–7 h Pregnancy category C	*Range:* 900–1800 mg/d *Start:* 300 mg po 3 × daily; titrate up to 1800 mg/d in divided doses (doses up to 3600 mg/d have been used)	*Use:* Partial seizures. *Off label:* Bipolar disorder and chronic pain *CSE:* Drowsiness, ataxia, confusion, depression; may also cause dizziness, hostility, vertigo, hypertension, anorexia	Use cautiously; especially with renal impairment (↓ dose and/or ↑ dosing interval).	Anticonvulsant/ mood stabilizer *Caution:* Renal impairment (↓ dose). Discontinuation requires at least a wk; should be done gradually; dosages no more than 12 h apart. Risk of CNS depression with alcohol, opioids, other CNS depressants.

Continued

Psychotropic Drugs A – Z (Alphabetical Listing)—cont'd

Generic (Trade)	Dose Range/ Adult Daily Dose	Use/Common Side Effects (CSE)	Geriatric & Dose Considerations	Classification Assessment Cautions
Haloperidol (Haldol, *Apo-Haloperidol*) Haloperidol decanoate T½ = 21–24 h Protein Binding = 90% Pregnancy category C	*Range:* 1–100 mg/d *Haloperidol:* 0.5–5 mg po 2–3 × d (to 100 mg/d). *Decanoate (IM):* 10–15 times the oral dose; given monthly	*Use:* Psychotic disorders, aggressive states, schizophrenia *CSE:* EPS, blurred vision, constipation, dry mouth/eyes, NMS, SEIZURES	*Dosage reduction required:* 0.5–2 mg po two × daily; increasing gradually; *Caution:* CV/ diabetes, BPH. ↑ mortality in dementia-related psychosis in the elderly.	Antipsychotic [Conventional] *Monitor* BP, pulse, respiration, akathisia, EPS, tardive dyskinesia, NMS (report immediately). Perform CBC w diff, LFTs, eye exams periodically. Avoid alcohol/CNS depressants. *Caution:* Toxic encephalopathy w haloperidol + lithium
Hydroxyzine (Atarax, Vistaril, Apo-Hydroxyzine, Novohydroxyzin) T½ = 3 h Pregnancy category C	Range: 100–400 mg/d 25–100 mg po 4 × daily (do not exceed 600 mg/d).	Use: Anxiety, pruritis, preop sedation CSE: Drowsiness, dry mouth, pain at IM site	Dosage reduction; severe hepatic disease; at ↑ risk for falls and CNS effects. *Monitor* for drowsiness, agitation, sedation.	Antianxiety/ sedative/hypnotic *Contraindicated* in pregnancy. Use cautiously severe hepatic dysfunction. Avoid alcohol/ CNS depressants.

Continued

Psychotropic Drugs A – Z (Alphabetical Listing)—cont'd

Generic (Trade)	Dose Range/ Adult Daily Dose	Use/Common Side Effects (CSE)	Geriatric & Dose Considerations	Classification Assessment Cautions
Iloperidone (Fanapt) Protein binding = 95% Pregnancy Category C	Recommended target dosage is 12–24 mg/day administered twice daily. Start 1 mg twice daily and titrate up slowly to avoid orthostatic hypotension.	*Use:* Acute treatment of schizophrenia *CSE:* dizziness, dry mouth, fatigue, nasal congestion, orthostatic hypotension, somnolence, tachycardia, weight gain	Clinical trials did not include sufficient enough pts 65 y or older for comparison to younger adults. *Great caution* because of dizziness, orthostatic hypotension. *Warning:* ↑ mortality in elderly with dementia-related psychosis	*Caution:* Prolongs QT interval and may be associated with arrhythmia and sudden death—consider other antipsychotics first. Avoid use in combination with other drugs that prolong QTc; *Monitor* for hyperglycemia, DM, weight gain, TD, NMS, suicidality early on and throughout Rx. Beware of orthostatic hypotension, syncope. Cases of PRIAPISM have been reported. Not recommended for hepatic impairment. Beware multiple drug interactions.

Continued

Psychotropic Drugs A – Z (Alphabetical Listing)—cont'd

Generic (Trade)	Dose Range/ Adult Daily Dose	Use/Common Side Effects (CSE)	Geriatric & Dose Considerations	Classification **Assessment Cautions**
Imipramine (Tofranil, *Apo-Imipramine*) T½ = 8–16 h Protein binding = 89–95% Pregnancy category C	*Range:* 30–300 mg/d 25–50 mg po 3–4 × daily (not to exceed 300 mg/d)	*Use:* Depression *CSE:* Blurred vision, dry eyes, dry mouth, sedation, constipation, hypotension, ARRHYTHMIAS	25 mg po hs initially, up to 100 mg/d, divided doses; Use cautiously in elderly, preexisting CV disease (*monitor* ECGs), BPH	Antidepressant [TCA] *Monitor* ECGs in heart disease; also BP and pulse. *Contraindicated:* Concurrent MAOIs; avoid use with SSRIs, or clonidine
Lamotrigine (Lamictal) T½ = 25.4 h (on lamotrigine alone) Pregnancy category C	*Range:* 75–250 mg/d *Bipolar pt not on CBZ/VA:* Start 25 mg/d po × 2 wk, then 50 mg/d × 2 wk, then 100 mg/d × 1 wk, then 200 mg/d	*Use:* Partial seizures, bipolar I disorder maintenance *CSE:* Nausea, vomiting, dizziness, headache, ataxia photosensitivity, rash, STEVENS-JOHNSON SYNDROME (SJS)	May cause dizziness/ drowsiness; *Caution* with impaired renal/CV/ hepatic disease	Anticonvulsant/ mood stabilizer *Contrainidicated:* Lactation. *Caution:* Impaired renal/ cardiac/hepatic function, hx rash on lamotrigine. Avoid abrupt discontinuation. *Assess* for skin rash. **Sx of SJS:** Cough, FUO, mucosal lesions, rash; ***stop lamotrigine***

Continued

Psychotropic Drugs A – Z (Alphabetical Listing)—cont'd

Generic (Trade)	Dose Range/ Adult Daily Dose	Use/Common Side Effects (CSE)	Geriatric & Dose Considerations	Classification Assessment Cautions
Lithium (Eskalith, Eskalith CR, Lithobid, Lithonate, Lithotabs, *Carbolith, Duralith*) T½ = 20–27 h Pregnancy category D	*Acute mania:* 1800–2400 mg/d; *Maintenance:* 300–1200 mg/d. *Start:* 300–600 mg po 3 × daily; usual maintenance: 300 mg 3–4 × daily. *Slow release*: 200–300 mg po 3 × daily to start, up to 1800 mg/d (divided doses); *Extended release:* 300–600 mg po 3 × daily to start	*Use:* Bipolar disorder: Acute manic episodes; prophylaxis against recurrence *CSE:* Fatigue, headache, impaired memory, ECG changes, bloating, diarrhea, nausea, abdominal pain, leukocytosis, polyuria, acne, hypothyroidism, tremors, weight gain, SEIZURES, ARRHYTHMIAS	Initial dose reduction recommended; *caution* w CV/renal/ thyroid disease, diabetes mellitus	Antimanic/mood stabilizer Serum lithium levels: *Acute mania:* 1.0–1.5 mEq/L; *Maintenance:* 0.6–1.2 mEq/L. Narrow therapeutic range; *Signs of toxicity:* vomiting, diarrhea, slurred speech, drowsiness, ↓ coordination. Li ↓ thyroid function (hypothyroidism)/ renal changes. *Monitor* thyroid/ kidney function, WBC w diff, electrolytes, glucose, ECG, weight (also BMI). *Caution:* Toxic encephalopathy w haloperidol + lithium

Continued

Psychotropic Drugs A – Z (Alphabetical Listing)—cont'd

Generic (Trade)	Dose Range/ Adult Daily Dose	Use/Common Side Effects (CSE)	Geriatric & Dose Considerations	Classification Assessment Cautions
Lorazepam (Ativan, *Apo-Lorazepam*) T½ = 10–16 h Schedule IV Pregnancy category D	*Range:* 2–6 mg/d (up to 10 mg/d); 1–3 mg po 2–3 × daily; *Insomnia:* 2–4 mg po hs	*Use:* Anxiety, insomnia *CSE:* Dizziness, drowsiness, lethargy; rapid IV: APNEA, CARDIAC ARREST	Dosage reduction; *Caution:* hepatic/ renal/ pulmonary impairment; more susceptible to CNS effects and increased risk for falls	Antianxiety/sedative/ hypnotic [benzo] *Contraindicated:* Comatose or CNS depression, pregnancy, lactation, glaucoma. *Caution:* In hepatic/renal/ pulmonary impairment/drug abuse
Loxapine (Loxitane, *Loxapac*) T½ = 5 h/ 12–19 h Pregnancy category C	*Range:* 20–250 mg/d *Start:* 10 mg po 2 × daily, ↑ until psychotic symptom improvement.	*Use:* Schizophrenia (second line Rx); *Off label*: other psychotic disorders, bipolar. *CSE:* Drowsiness, orthostatic hypotension, ataxia, constipation, nausea, blurred vision	*Evaluate/monitor* for confusion, orthostatic hypotension, sedation, ↓ dose; at risk for falls; ↑ mortality in elderly with dementia-related psychosis	Antipsychotic [Conventional] *Contraindicated:* Severe CNS depression/coma. *Caution:* Parkinson's, bone marrow suppression, cardiac, renal, respiratory disease; sedating, *Monitor* for EPS, NMS, TD, BMI, FBS, lipids

Continued

Psychotropic Drugs A – Z (Alphabetical Listing)—cont'd

Generic (Trade)	Dose Range/ Adult Daily Dose	Use/Common Side Effects (CSE)	Geriatric & Dose Considerations	Classification Assessment Cautions
Lurasidone HCL (Latuda) T½ = 18 h Protein binding = 99% Pregnancy category B	Starting dose 40 mg po once daily, up to 80 mg once daily; take with food	*Use:* Schizophrenia *CSE:* somnolence, akathisia, nausea, parkinsonism, agitation	*Caution:* Start with lowest dose; *monitor* for somnolence, dizziness, hypotension, cognitive/motor impairment *Warning:* ↑ mortality in elderly with dementia-related psychosis	Antipsychotic [Atypical] *Caution:* Do not use in combination w strong CYP3A4 inhibitors (ketoconazole) or inducers (rifampin). Adjust dose for moderate CYP3A4 inhibitors (diltiazem). *Monitor* for hyperglycemia, DM, weight gain. Beware of orthostatic hypotension, syncope, seizures. Renal/hepatic impairment: adjust dose. *Monitor* for suicidality early on and throughout Rx.

Continued

Psychotropic Drugs A – Z (Alphabetical Listing)—cont'd

Generic (Trade)	Dose Range/ Adult Daily Dose	Use/Common Side Effects (CSE)	Geriatric & Dose Considerations	Classification **Assessment Cautions**
Mirtazapine (Remeron, Remeron Soltabs) T½ = 20–40 h Protein binding = 85% Pregnancy category C	*Range:* 15–45 mg/d *Start:* 15 mg/d po hs, increase q 1–2 wk up to 45 mg/d	*Use:* Major depressive disorder; *Off label:* Panic disorder, GAD, PTSD *CSE:* Drowsiness, constipation, dry mouth, increased appetite, weight gain	Lower dose; use *cautiously* w hepatic/renal disease	Antidepressant [Tetracyclic] *Contraindicated:* Concurrent MAOI therapy; *caution* w hx seizures, suicide attempt. Closely *monitor* for suicidality/safety not determined in children, lactation, pregnancy. Periodic CBCs, LFTs.
Molindone (Moban) T½ = 1.5 h Pregnancy category unknown	*Range:* 15–225 mg/d *Start:* 50–75 mg/d po, increase at 4 d intervals (up to 225 mg)	*Use:* Psychotic disorders, schizophrenia *CSE:* Sedation, drowsiness, constipation, weight gain, blurred vision	Initial ↓ dose; *Caution* w diabetes, BPH, respiratory disease; increased risk for falls (sedation/ orthostatic hypotension); ↑ mortality in dementia-related psychosis	Antipsychotic *Contraindicated* w CNS depression. *Monitor* for EPS, NMS, and TD. *Caution* with cardiac, renal, hepatic, respiratory disease. *Monitor* for BMI, FBS, and lipids.

Continued

Psychotropic Drugs A – Z (Alphabetical Listing)—cont'd

Generic (Trade)	Dose Range/ Adult Daily Dose	Use/Common Side Effects (CSE)	Geriatric & Dose Considerations	Classification Assessment Cautions
MAOIs: Phenelzine (Nardil) Tranylcypromine (Parnate) Isocarboxazid (Marplan) T½ = Unknown [See selegiline patch] Pregnancy category C	**Phenelzine:** *Range:* 45–90 mg/d *Start:* 15 mg po 3 × daily and increase to 60–90 mg/d. **Tranylcypromine:** *Range:* 30–60 mg/d *Start:* 30 mg/d po divided dose (AM/PM) up to 60 mg/d. **Isocarboxazid:** *Range:* 20–60 mg/d *Start:* 10 mg/d po, increasing every few days (up to 60 mg/d in 2–4 divided doses)	*Use:* Atypical depression, panic disorder; other Rx ineffective or not tolerated *CSE:* Dizziness, headaches, insomnia, restlessness, blurred vision, arrythmias, orthostatic hypotension, diarrhea, SEIZURES, HYPERTENSIVE CRISIS	Use cautiously, titrate slowly, ↑ risk of adverse reactions	Antidepressant Potentially fatal reactions with other antidepressants (SSRIs, TCAs, etc). 5-wk washout w fluoxetine. *Must follow MAOI diet (foods high in tyramine) to avoid hypertensive crisis (emergency)* [See MAOI diet in Drug-Lab Tab]; hypertensive crisis from caffeine; also amphetamines, levadopa, dopamine, epinephrine, reserpine, and others. Avoid opioids (meperidine).

Continued

Psychotropic Drugs A – Z (Alphabetical Listing)—cont'd

Generic (Trade)	Dose Range/ Adult Daily Dose	Use/Common Side Effects (CSE)	Geriatric & Dose Considerations	Classification **Assessment Cautions**
Nadolol (Corgard; Syn-Nadolol) T½ = 10–24 h Pregnancy category C	40 mg/d po (up to 240 mg)	*Use:* Tremors, akathisia *CSE:* Fatigue, impotence, ARRYTHMIAS, CHF, BRADYCARDIA, PULMONARY EDEMA	Initial dose reduction recommended; increased sensitivity to beta blockers	Antianginal; beta blocker *Contraindicated:* CV diseases (CHF, bradycardia, heart block, etc.); *renal impairment:* ↑ dosing intervals
Nefazodone (Serzone*) Pregnancy category C *Wthdrawn from North American market	200–600 mg/d po	*Use:* Depression *CSE:* Insomnia, dizziness, drowsiness, HEPATIC FAILURE; HEPATIC TOXICITY	Initiate lower dose; HEPATIC FAILURE; HEPATIC TOXICITY	Antidepressant Serzone has been withdrawn from the North American market for *rare but serious liver failure;* generic is still available

Continued

Psychotropic Drugs A – Z (Alphabetical Listing)—cont'd

Generic (Trade)	Dose Range/ Adult Daily Dose	Use/Common Side Effects (CSE)	Geriatric & Dose Considerations	Classification Assessment Cautions
Nortriptyline (Pamelor, Aventyl) T½ = 18–28 h Protein binding = 92% Pregnancy category D	*Range:* 75–150 mg/d *Start:* 25 mg po 3–4 × daily up to 150 mg/d	*Use:* Major depressive disorder; *Off label:* Chronic neurogenic pain, anxiety, insomnia *CSE:* Drowsiness, fatigue, blurred vision, dry eyes/mouth, hypotension, constipation, ARRYTHMIAS	*Susceptible to side effects:* ↓ Dose: 30–50 mg/d po in divided doses; *Caution* w BPH, CV disease; *Monitor* ECGs in elderly.	Antidepressant [TCA] *Contraindicated* in narrow-angle glaucoma. Potential fatal reaction with MAOIs. *Monitor* ECGs w heart disease.
Olanzapine (Zyprexa, Zyprexa Zydis, Zyprexa Intramuscular) T½ = 21–54 h Protein binding = 93% Pregnancy category C [Zyprexa Relprevv: Extended release IM; up to 4 wk]	*Range:* 5–20 mg/d **Schizophrenia**: *Start:* 5–10 mg po/d (not to exceed 20 mg/d) **Bipolar**: *Start:* 10–15 mg/d po (not to exceed 20 mg/d); *IM (acute agitation):* 5–10 mg, may repeat in 2 h/4 h	*Use:* Schizophrenia, psychotic disorders; Bipolar: Acute mania; mixed episodes; long-term maintenance *CSE:* Agitation, dizziness, sedation, orthostatic hypotension, constipation, weight gain, NMS, SEIZURES	Dosage reduction may be needed; reduce dosage for debilitated or non-smoking females ≥65: *start* at 5 mg/d po. *Caution* w CV, CVA, BPH, hepatic disease. ↑ mortality in elderly with dementia-related psychosis	Antipsychotic [Atypical] *Monitor* for treatment-emergent diabetes (serum glucose, BMI), akathisia, EPS, NMS; perform CBCs, LFTs, eye exams. *Monitor* BP, pulse, respiratory rate, ECG.

Continued

Psychotropic Drugs A – Z (Alphabetical Listing)—cont'd

Generic (Trade)	Dose Range/ Adult Daily Dose	Use/Common Side Effects (CSE)	Geriatric & Dose Considerations	Classification Assessment Cautions
Olanzapine and fluoxetine HCl (Symbyax) Olanzapine T½ = 21–54 h Protein binding = 93% Fluoxetine T½ = 1–3 d (norfluoxetine: 5–7 d) Protein binding = 94.5% Pregnancy category C	*Dosing options:* 6/25, 6/50, 12/25, 12/50 mg/d *Efficacy:* fluoxetine 6–12 mg and olanzapine 25–50 mg. Start 6/25 mg once daily po in evening	*Use:* Bipolar depressive disorder *CSE:* Drowsiness, weight gain, dry mouth, diarrhea, increased appetite, tremor, sore throat, weakness, NMS, TD	Start with 6/25 mg/d, especially if hypotensive or hepatic impairment or slow metabolism; ↑ mortality in dementia-related psychosis in the elderly	Antipsychotic/ antidepressant Same as olanzapine and fluoxetine

Continued

Psychotropic Drugs A – Z (Alphabetical Listing)—cont'd

Generic (Trade)	Dose Range/ Adult Daily Dose	Use/Common Side Effects (CSE)	Geriatric & Dose Considerations	Classification Assessment Cautions
Oxazepam (Serax, *Apo-Oxazepam*) T½ = 5–15 h Protein binding = 97% Schedule IV Pregnancy category D	*Range:* 30–120 mg/d *Anxiety:* 10–30 mg po 3–4 × daily *Sedative/ alcohol withdrawal:* 15–30 mg po 3–4 × daily	*Use:* Anxiety, alcohol withdrawal *CSE:* Dizziness, drowsiness, hangover, impaired memory, blurred vision, constipation, nausea	↓ *dose:* Start 5 mg po 1–2 × daily, may increase as needed; caution w hepatic, severe COPD disease; ↑ risk for falls	Antianxiety/ sedative/hypnotic [benzo] *Contraindicated:* CNS depression, coma, narrow-angle glaucoma, pregnancy, lactation *Caution:* Hepatic dysfunction; monitor CBCs, LFTs, avoid alcohol
Paliperidone (Invega) Major active metabolite of risperidone Protein binding = 74% Pregnancy category C	*Range:* 3–12 mg/d Usual dose: 6 mg/d po extended-release tab in AM (once daily dosing)	*Use:* Schizophrenia *CSE:* Somnolence, orthostatic hypotension, akathisia, EPS, parkinsonism	*Caution* w decreased renal function; moderate to severe renal impairment (dose: 3 mg/d); ↑ mortality with dementia-related psychosis	Antipsychotic [Atypical] Causes ↑ in QT interval; avoid drugs that prolong QT int (e.g., quinidine). *Monitor* BMI, FBS, and lipids.

Continued

Psychotropic Drugs A – Z (Alphabetical Listing)—cont'd

Generic (Trade)	Dose Range/ Adult Daily Dose	Use/Common Side Effects (CSE)	Geriatric & Dose Considerations	Classification Assessment Cautions
Paroxetine HCL (Paxil, Paxil CR); **paroxetine mesylate**: Pevexa $T½$ = 24 h Protein binding = 95% Pregnancy category D	*Range:* 10–60 mg/d; *CR:* 12.5–75 mg/d. Depression*: Start* 20 mg po q AM (may increase by 10 mg/d at weekly intervals) *CR: Start* 25 mg po once daily, may increase weekly by 1.25 mg, up to 62.5 mg/d	*Use: Paxil/CR/Pevexa*: Depression, panic disorder; *Paxil/Pevexa:* OCD, GAD; *Paxil:* PTSD; *Paxil CR:* PMDD; *Paxil/CR:* Social anxiety disorder. *CSE:* Anxiety, dizziness, drowsiness, dry mouth, headache, insomnia, nausea, constipation, diarrhea, weakness, ejaculatory disturbance, sweating, tremor	↓ *dose:* start 10 mg/d po, up to 40 mg/d; *CR:* Start 12.5 mg po daily, up to 50 mg/d. *Caution* w hepatic, renal impairment.	Antidepressant/ antianxiety [SSRI] *Caution:* Hepatic, renal, seizure disorders/ pregnancy/ lactation. *Withdrawal syndrome:* Do not stop abruptly. *Peds/Adol (18–24 y):* ↑ risk for suicide; weigh risks vs benefits; *Closely monitor* for suicidality (see FDA warning, end of tab)

Continued

Psychotropic Drugs A – Z (Alphabetical Listing)—cont'd

Generic (Trade)	Dose Range/ Adult Daily Dose	Use/Common Side Effects (CSE)	Geriatric & Dose Considerations	Classification Assessment Cautions
Phenobarbital (Luminal, *Ancalixir)* T½ = 2–6 d Schedule IV Pregnancy category D	*Range:* 30–320 mg/d *Sedation:* 30–120 mg/d po/IM (divided doses) *Hypnotic:* 120–320 mg hs (PO, SC, IV, IM)	*Use:* Sedative/ hypnotic (short term) *CSE:* Hangover, drowsiness, excitation	Use cautiously; ↓ dose; hepatic/ renal disease.	Sedative/hypnotic [Barbiturate] *Life-threatening side effects:* ANGIOEDEMA, SERUM SICKNESS, LARYNGOSPASM (IV). *IV:* Monitor BP, pulse, respiratory status. Resuscitation equipment available.
Pimozide (Orap) T½ = 29–111 h Protein binding = 99% Pregnancy category C	*Range:* 2–10 mg/d Start 1–2 mg/d po, increase as needed every other day	*Use:* Tourette's, psychosis (2nd line Rx) *CSE:* Orthostatic hypotension, palpitations, QT prolongation, drowsiness, dizziness, blurred vision	Moderately sedating; *caution* in Parkinson's, arrhythmias, cerebrovascular, cardiovascular disease; may cause orthostatic hypotension; ↑ mortality in elderly with dementia-related psychosis	Antipsychotic [Conventional] *Contraindicated:* CNS depression, prolonged QT syndrome, dysrhythmias. *Caution* in respiratory, CV, hepatic, renal disease. *Assess* for EPS, TD, akathisia, NMS, BMI, FBS, and lipids.

Continued

Psychotropic Drugs A – Z (Alphabetical Listing)—cont'd

Generic (Trade)	Dose Range/ Adult Daily Dose	Use/Common Side Effects (CSE)	Geriatric & Dose Considerations	Classification **Assessment** **Cautions**
Propranolol (Inderal, *Apo-propranolol*) T½ = 3.4–6 h Protein binding = 93% Pregnancy category C	*Tremors:* 80–120 mg/d po (up to 320 mg/d) *Akathisia:* 30–120 mg/d po	*Use:* Essential tremor, anxiety, akathisia *CSE:* Fatigue, weakness, impotence, ARRHYTHMIAS, BRADYCARDIA, CHF, PULMONARY EDEMA	↓ dose (elderly have increased sensitivity to beta blockers); renal, hepatic, pulmonary disease, diabetes	Antianginal/beta blocker *Contraindicated:* Heart block, CHF, bradycardia. *Monitor* BP, pulse, & for orthostatic hypotension. *Abrupt withdrawal:* life-threatening arrhythmias.

Continued

Psychotropic Drugs A – Z (Alphabetical Listing)—cont'd

Generic (Trade)	Dose Range/ Adult Daily Dose	Use/Common Side Effects (CSE)	Geriatric & Dose Considerations	Classification Assessment Cautions
Quetiapine (Seroquel) T½ = 6 h [Seroquel XR—once daily dosing] Pregnancy category C	Range: 150–800 mg/d *Schizophrenia:* Start 25 mg po 2 × daily, gradually increase to 300–400/800 mg/d. *Bipolar mania:* Start 100 mg/d po 2 divided doses, up to 800 mg/d (incremental) *Bipolar depression:* Start 50 mg, up to 300 mg by day 4.	*Use:* Schizophrenia, Bipolar I mania: (monotherapy and adjunct to lithium/ divalproex (bipolar maintenance); *Bipolar I and II*: acute depressive episodes *CSE:* Dizziness, headache, somnolence, weight gain, NMS, SEIZURES	May require dose reduction; use cautiously in Alzheimer's, pts ≥65 y, & hx seizures. *Warning:* ↑ mortality in elderly with dementia-related psychosis. Also *caution* w CV/ hepatic disease.	Antipsychotic [Atypical]/mood stabilizer *Contraindicated:* Lactation. *Caution* in CV disease; cerebrovascular disease, dehydration. *Monitor* for EPS, NMS. *Monitor* BP (hypotension), pulse during dose titration. [See product prescribing info for dosing for adjunctive therapies.]

Continued

Psychotropic Drugs A – Z (Alphabetical Listing)—cont'd

Generic (Trade)	Dose Range/ Adult Daily Dose	Use/Common Side Effects (CSE)	Geriatric & Dose Considerations	Classification Assessment Cautions
Ramelteon (Rozerem) [melatonin receptor agonist] T½ = 1–2.6 h; M-II metabolite 2–5 h Protein binding = 82% Pregnancy category C	*Adult dose:* 8 mg po within 30 min of sleep; do not administer with high-fat meal	*Use:* Insomnia (difficulty with sleep onset) *CSE:* Somnolence, dizziness, nausea, fatigue, headache *FDA warning:* Risk of severe allergic reaction and complex sleep-related behaviors (e.g., sleep-driving)	As with any drug that causes somnolence and dizziness, use with caution	Sedative/hypnotic *Contraindicated:* Severe liver disease and fluvoxamine (CYP 1A2 inhibitor). *Interactions* with rifampin and azole antifungals (ketoconazole). Effect on reproductive hormones in adults (↓ testosterone, ↑ prolactin). Avoid alcohol. In pregnancy, benefit must outweigh risk. *Report:* ↓ menses, galactorrhea, ↓ libido, ↓ fertility.

Continued

Psychotropic Drugs A – Z (Alphabetical Listing)—cont'd

Generic (Trade)	Dose Range/ Adult Daily Dose	Use/Common Side Effects (CSE)	Geriatric & Dose Considerations	Classification Assessment Cautions
Risperidone (Risperdal, Risperdal M-Tab, Risperdal Consta Long-acting Injection) T½ = *Metabolizers:* 3 h (9-hydroxy-risperidone, 21 h) *Poor metabolizers:* 20 h (9-hydroxy-risperidone, 30 h) Pregnancy category C	*Range:* 4–12 mg/d Dosing may be once/d (↑ risk of EPS w dose > 6 mg) *Schizophrenia:* Start 1 mg po 2 × daily, ↑ to 3 mg 2 × daily (up to 16 mg/d). *IM:* 25 mg q 2 wk, may ↑ 37.5/50 mg. *Bipolar Mania:* 2–3 mg/d po (range: 1–5 mg/d)	*Use:* Schizophrenia; bipolar: mania, acute or mixed; new indication: irritability associated with autism *CSE:* EPS (akathisia), dizziness, aggression, insomnia, sedation, dry mouth, pharyngitis, cough, visual disturbances, itching, skin rash, constipation, diarrhea, libido, weight gain/loss, NMS	*Warning:* ↑ mortality in elderly with dementia-related psychosis *Caution:* Renal/hepatic disease/CV disease. *Bipolar mania:* Start 0.5 mg po 2 × daily, up to 1.5 mg 2 × daily (gradually increase weekly if necessary at small increments)	Antipsychotic [Atypical] *Caution:* Renal/hepatic impairment. Dosing may be once daily or bid and increments should be small (1 mg). Maximal effect seen with 4–8 mg/d, and doses above 6 mg/d not more efficacious, and with ↑ risk of EPS. *Monitor* BP, pulse during titration: may cause tachycardia, hypotension, QT prolongation. Establish oral dosing tolerance before using IM. *Monitor* BMI, FBS, and lipids.

Continued

Psychotropic Drugs A – Z (Alphabetical Listing)—cont'd

Generic (Trade)	Dose Range/ Adult Daily Dose	Use/Common Side Effects (CSE)	Geriatric & Dose Considerations	Classification Assessment Cautions
Selegiline Patch (Emsam) [MAOI] First transdermal patch delivering medication systemically over 24 h period. Protein binding = 90% over a 2–500 ng/mL concentration range. Pregnancy category C	*Range:* 6 mg/24 h to 12 mg/24 h *Recommended starting and target dose:* 6 mg/24 h	*Use:* Major depressive disorder *CSE:* Mild skin reaction/redness at patch site. D/C if redness continues for several hours after patch removal; hypotension HYPERTENSION	Patients 50 yr and older at higher risk for rash	Antidepressant *With doses above 6 mg/24 h, must follow MAOI diet (foods high in tyramine).* Hypertensive crisis is an emergency. *Contraindicated:* Amphetamines, pseudoephedrine, etc; other selegiline products (Eldepryl). *Monitor* BP, also for headache, nausea, stiff neck, palpitations. Close monitoring of children for suicidality. Read full prescribing information.

Continued

Psychotropic Drugs A – Z (Alphabetical Listing)—cont'd

Generic (Trade)	Dose Range/ Adult Daily Dose	Use/Common Side Effects (CSE)	Geriatric & Dose Considerations	Classification Assessment Cautions
Sertraline (Zoloft) T½ = 24 h Protein binding = 98% Pregnancy category C	*Range:* 50–200 mg/d *Depression/OCD: Start:* 50 mg/d po AM or PM, may ↑ slowly/weekly to 200 mg/d *Panic disorder:* Start: 25 mg/d po, up to 50 mg/d *PTSD/SAD:* Start: 25 mg/d po (to 200 mg/d)	*Use:* Depression, panic disorder, OCD, PTSD, social anxiety disorder (SAD), PMDD; *Off label:* GAD *CSE:* Drowsiness, dizziness, headache, fatigue, insomnia, nausea, diarrhea, dry mouth, sexual dysfunction, sweating, tremor	Caution with drowsiness, hepatic/renal impairment; start with lower dose.	Antidepressant [SSRI] *Contraindicated:* Concurrent Pimozide or MAOIs (serious fatal reactions), need 14 d washout period. Do not use with St. John's wort or SAMe. *Caution*: Hepatic/renal/ pregnancy/lactation/seizures/ hx mania. *Peds/Adol: May increase the risk of suicidal thinking and behavior and must be closely monitored.*

Continued

Psychotropic Drugs A – Z (Alphabetical Listing)—cont'd

Generic (Trade)	Dose Range/ Adult Daily Dose	Use/Common Side Effects (CSE)	Geriatric & Dose Considerations	Classification Assessment Cautions
Thioridazine* (Mellaril, Mellaril-S, *Apo-thioridazine, Novo-Ridazine*) T½ = 21–24 h Protein binding = ≥90% Pregnancy category C [*Mellaril discontinued worldwide for serious side effects; generic still available]	*Range:* 150–800 mg/d *Start:* 50–100 mg po tid, increase gradually up to 800 mg/d	*Use:* Schizophrenia *CSE:* Sedation, blurred vision, dry eyes, hypotension, constipation, dry mouth, photosensitivity NMS, ARRYTHMIAS QTC PROLONGATION, AGRANULOCYTOSIS	Use cautiously, at risk for EPS/CNS adverse effects. ↑ risk for falls (sedation/ dehydration/ hypotension); *Caution* with CV disease, BPH. Be especially careful with debilitated patients; ↑ mortality in elderly with dementia-related psychosis	Antipsychotic [Conventional] *Contraindicated:* QTc interval >450 msec; agents that prolong QTc interval; also, narrow-angle glaucoma, bone marrow depression, severe liver or cardiovascular disease. *Monitor* BP, pulse, resp, and ECGs, CBCs, eye exams. *Monitor* for agranulocytosis; occurs between 4–10 wk of Rx. *Assess* for NMS, TD, akathisia.

Continued

Psychotropic Drugs A – Z (Alphabetical Listing)—cont'd

Generic (Trade)	Dose Range/ Adult Daily Dose	Use/Common Side Effects (CSE)	Geriatric & Dose Considerations	Classification Assessment Cautions
Topiramate (Topamax) T½ = 21 h Pregnancy category C	*Range:* 50–400 mg/d (maximum dose: 1600 mg/d) *Start:* 50 mg/d po, increase 50 mg/wk up to 200 mg bid	*Use:* Seizures, migraines; *Off label:* bipolar, treatment-resistant *CSE:* Dizziness, drowsiness, impaired memory/concentration, nervousness, diplopia, nystagmus, nausea, weight loss, ataxia, paresthesias, INCREASED SEIZURES, SUICIDE ATTEMPT	Adjust dose ↓ for renal/hepatic impairment. Dosage reduction recommended if CCr <70 mL/min/ 1.73 m^2 for adults and geriatric population	Anticonvulsant/ mood stabilizer *Contraindicated:* Lactation. *Topiramate* has not been shown to be as effective as monotherapy in bipolar disorder, may be efficacious as adjunctive treatment. Concomitant use with valproic acid associated with hyperammonemia (with or without encephalopathy). *Monitor* for alterations in LOC, cognitive function, lethargy, vomiting.

Continued

Psychotropic Drugs A – Z (Alphabetical Listing)—cont'd

Generic (Trade)	Dose Range/ Adult Daily Dose	Use/Common Side Effects (CSE)	Geriatric & Dose Considerations	Classification Assessment Cautions
Trazodone (Oleptro, Trialodine, Trazon) T½ = 5–9 h Protein binding = 89%–95% Pregnancy category C [Desyrel discontinued]	*Range:* 150–400 mg/d (hospitalized up to 600 mg/d) *Depression:* 50 mg po tid (150 mg/d), up to 400 mg/d (titrate 50 mg every 4 d). *Insomnia:* 25–100 mg hs *Oleptro:* Start 150 mg once daily; max. dose 375 mg/d	*Use:* Major depression. *Off label:* Insomnia *CSE:* Drowsiness, hypotension, dry mouth, PRIAPISM; may also experience confusion, dizziness, insomnia, nightmares, palpitations, impotence, myalgia	Reduce dose initially. *Start:* 75 mg/d po in divided doses, increase every 4 d; titrate slowly; *caution* w CV, hepatic, renal disease. Observe elderly for drowsiness & hypotension; caution about slow positional changes	Antidepressant/ sedative PRIAPISM (prolonged erection): Medical emergency; avoid alcohol, concomitant use with fluoxetine, opioids, and drugs that inhibit and induce the CYP3A4 enzyme system; also kava, valerian (↑ CNS depression), St. John's wort and SAMe (serotonin syndrome)

Continued

Psychotropic Drugs A – Z (Alphabetical Listing)—cont'd

Generic (Trade)	Dose Range/ Adult Daily Dose	Use/Common Side Effects (CSE)	Geriatric & Dose Considerations	Classification Assessment Cautions
Trihexyphenidyl (Artane, Artane Sequels, *Apo-Trihex*) $T\frac{1}{2} = 3.7$ h Pregnancy category C	*Range:* 6–10 mg/d (up to 15 mg/d) *Start:* 1–2 mg/d po; ↑ by 2 mg every 3–5 d *Sequels (ER):* q 12 h *after* dose is determined w tabs/elixir Monitor for decreased signs & symptoms of parkinsonian syndrome: ↓ tremors/rigidity	*Use:* Parkinson's, drug-induced parkinsonism and EPS *CSE:* Dizziness, nervousness, drowsiness, blurred vision, mydriasis, dry mouth, nausea; may also experience orthostatic hypotension, tachycardia, and urinary hesitancy	*Caution w elderly:* Causes drowsiness/ dizziness (↑ risk-adverse reactions); BPH, chronic renal, hepatic, CV, pulmonary disease	Antiparkinsonian agent *Contraindicated:* Glaucoma, thyrotoxicosis, tachycardia (due to cardiac insufficiency), acute hemorrhage. Alcohol intolerance (Elixir only). Additive effects with anticholinergic drugs and CNS depressants.

Continued

Psychotropic Drugs A – Z (Alphabetical Listing)—cont'd

Generic (Trade)	Dose Range/ Adult Daily Dose	Use/Common Side Effects (CSE)	Geriatric & Dose Considerations	Classification **Assessment Cautions**
Venlafaxine (Effexor, Effexor XR) T½ = venlafaxine: 3–5 h; O-desmethylvenlafaxine (ODV) 9–11 h Pregnancy category C	*Range:* 75–225 mg/d; do not exceed 375 mg/d *Start:* 75 mg/d po (2–3 divided doses), up to 225 mg/d (divided doses) (do not exceed 375 mg/d). *XR:* 37.5–75 mg po once daily; increase q 4 d up to 225 mg	*Use:* Major depression, generalized anxiety disorder (XR) and social anxiety disorder (XR) *CSE:* Anxiety, abnormal dreams, dizziness, insomnia, nervousness, visual disturbances, anorexia, dry mouth, weight loss, sexual dysfunction, ecchymoses (bruising), SEIZURES	Use cautiously with CV disease (hypertension); reduce dose in renal/hepatic impairment	Antidepressant [SNRI] *Caution* with preexisting hypertension. *Monitor* blood pressure (risk of sustained hypertension [treatment emergent]); may be dose-related. Concurrent MAOI therapy *contraindicated.* Avoid alcohol/CNS depressants.
Vilazodone HCl (Viibryd) T½ = 25 h Pregnancy category C	*Start:* 10 mg once daily; titrate to 40 mg/d	*Use:* Major depressive disorder *CSE:* diarrhea, N&V, insomnia	No dose adjustments needed; possible hyponatremia	Antidepressant [SSRI]; also 5 HT_{IA} receptor partial agonist; caution same as SSRIs

Continued

Psychotropic Drugs A – Z (Alphabetical Listing)—cont'd

Generic (Trade)	Dose Range/ Adult Daily Dose	Use/Common Side Effects (CSE)	Geriatric & Dose Considerations	Classification **Assessment** **Cautions**
Zaleplon (Sonata) T½ = Unknown Pregnancy category C	*Range:* 5–20 mg hs *Usual:* 10 mg po hs. Use no longer than 7–10 d	*Use:* Short-term insomnia, unable to initiate sleep *CSE:* Drowsiness, dizziness, anxiety, amnesia (see FDA warning, end of tab)	*Lower dose:* Start at 5 mg hs, to maximum of 10 mg po hs *Caution:* Mild/moderate hepatic impairment	Sedative/hypnotic *Contraindicated:* Severe hepatic impairment. *Avoid* other CNS depressants (alcohol, opioids, kava)
Ziprasidone (Geodon) T½ = po 7h; IM 2–5 h Protein binding = 99% Pregnancy category B	*Range:* 40–160 mg/d *Schizophrenia:* Start: 20 mg po bid, up to 80 mg bid *Mania:* Start: 40 mg po bid, up to 80 mg bid; *IM:* 10–20 mg prn (up to 40 mg/d)	*Use:* Schizophrenia, bipolar (manic and mixed), *IM:* acute agitation *CSE:* Dizziness, drowsiness, restlessness, nausea, constipation, diarrhea, PROLONGED QT INTERVAL, NMS	↓ Dose in elderly. *Contraindicated:* QT prolongation, *Caution* w CV/hepatic disease and CV drugs; >65 y; Alzheimer's dementia. Risk of falls. *Warning:* ↑ mortality in elderly with dementia-related psychosis	Antipsychotic [Atypical]/mood stabilizer Persistent QTc measurements >500: *D/C ziprasidone.* Evaluate palpitations, syncope. Agents (pimozide) that prolong QT interval are *contrainidicated. Avoid* CNS depressants. *Monitor* BP, pulse, ECG, and for EPS, NMS, and TD; also BMI, FBS, lipids.

Continued

Psychotropic Drugs A – Z (Alphabetical Listing)—cont'd

Generic (Trade)	Dose Range/ Adult Daily Dose	Use/Common Side Effects (CSE)	Geriatric & Dose Considerations	Classification **Assessment Cautions**
Zolpidem (Ambien, Ambien CR, Intermezzo) T½ = 2.5–2.6 h Schedule IV Pregnancy category B	*Range:* 5–10 mg hs *Usual:* 10 mg po hs; CR: 12.5 mg po hs *Intermezzo sublingual tab:* middle-of-night awakening; 1.75/3.5 mg once nightly	*Use:* Insomnia *CSE:* Amnesia, daytime drowsiness, "drugged" feeling, diarrhea, physical/ psychological dependence (see FDA warning, end of tab)	Initial ↓ dose; *geriatric or hepatic disease: Start:* 5 mg po hs, may increase to 10 mg; *CR:* 6.25 mg po hs	Sedative/hypnotic Caution in alcohol abuse and avoid use with CNS depressants. For short-term treatment of insomnia; after 2 wk, avoid abrupt withdrawal.

◎ **ALERT:** *Refer to the Physicians' Desk Reference or product insert (prescribing information) for complete and current drug information (dosages, warnings, indications, adverse effects, interactions, etc.) needed to make appropriate choices in the treatment of clients before administering any medications. Although every effort has been made to provide key information about medications and classes of drugs, such information is not and cannot be all-inclusive in a reference of this nature and should not be used for prescribing or administering of medications. Professional judgment, training, supervision, relevant references, and "current" drug information are critical to the appropriate selection, evaluation, and use of drugs, as well as the monitoring and management of clients and their medications.*

FDA WARNINGS (2007): *The US Food and Drug Administration wants all makers of* ***antidepressants*** *to include warnings about increased risk for suicidality in young adults ages 18–24 during initial treatment. The FDA also wants all manufacturers of* ***sedatives-hypnotics*** *to warn about possible severe allergic reactions as well as complex sleep-related behaviors, such as sleep-driving. If angioedema develops, seek treatment and do not use drug again.*
Complete drug monographs located at: http://davisplus.fadavis.com or see inside front cover.
Sources: Pedersen Pocket Psych Drugs 2010; Davis's Drug Guide 12th ed. 2011; prescribing information (product inserts).

Crisis/Suicide/Grief/Abuse

Crisis Intervention

Phases

I. Assessment – What caused the crisis, and what are the individual's responses to it?

II. Planning intervention – Explore individual's strengths, weaknesses, support systems, and coping skills in dealing with the crisis.

III. Intervention – Establish relationship, help understand event and explore feelings, and explore alternative coping strategies.

IV. Evaluation/reaffirmation – Evaluate outcomes/Plan for future/Evaluate need for follow-up (Aguilera 1998).

Prevention/Management of Assaultive Behaviors

Assessment of signs of anger is very important in prevention and in intervening *before anger escalates to assault/violence.*

Early Signs of Anger

- Muscular tension: clenched fist
- *Face:* furled brow, glaring eyes, tense mouth, clenched teeth, flushed face
- *Voice:* raised or lowered

If anger is not identified and recognized at the **preassaultive tension stage,** it can progress to aggressive behavior.

Anger Management Techniques

- Remain calm
- Help client recognize anger
- Find an outlet: verbal (talking) or physical (exercise)
- Help client accept angry feelings; *not acceptable to act on them*
- Do not touch an angry client
- Medication may be needed

Signs of Anger Escalation

- Verbal/physical threats
- Pacing/appears agitated
- Throwing objects
- Appears suspicious/disproportionate anger
- Acts of violence/hitting

Anger Management Techniques

- Speak in short command sentences: *Joe, calm down.*
- Never allow yourself to be cornered with an angry client; *always have an escape route* (open door behind you)
- *Request assistance of other staff*
- Medication may be needed; *offer voluntarily first*
- Restraints and/or seclusion may be needed *(see Use of Restraints in Basics tab)*
- Continue to *assess/reassess* (ongoing)
- When stabilized, *help client identify early signs/triggers of anger and alternatives* to prevent future anger/escalation

Suicide

Risk Factors Include:

- Mood disorders such as depression and bipolar disorder
- Substance abuse (dual diagnosis)
- Previous suicide attempt
- Loss – marital partner, partner, close relationship, job, health
- Expressed hopelessness or helplessness (does not see a future)
- Impulsivity/aggressiveness
- Family suicides, significant other or friend/peer suicide
- Isolation (lives alone/few friends, support relationships)
- Stressful life event
- Previous or current abuse (emotional/physical/sexual)
- Sexual identity crisis/conflict
- Available lethal method, such as a gun
- Legal issues/incarceration (USPHS, HHS 1999)

Suicide Assessment

- *Hopelessness* – a key element; client is unable to see a future or self in that future.
- *Speaks of suicide (suicidal ideation)* – important to ask client if he/she has thoughts of suicide; if so, should be considered suicidal.
- *Plan* – client is able to provide an exact method for ending life; must take seriously and consider immediacy of act.
- *Giving away possessions* – any actions such as giving away possessions, putting affairs in order (recent will), connecting anew with old friends/family members as a final goodbye.
- *Auditory hallucinations* – commanding client to kill self.
- *Lack of support network* – isolation, few friends or withdrawing from friends/support network.
- *Alcohol/other substance abuse* – drinking alone.
- *Previous suicide attempt or family history of suicide.*
- *Precipitating event* – death of a loved one; loss of a job, especially long-term job; holidays; tragedy; disaster.
- *Media* – suicide of a famous personality or local teenager (Rakel 2000).

CLINICAL PEARL – Do not confuse self-injurious behavior (cutting) with suicide attempts, although those who repeatedly cut themselves to relieve emotional pain could also attempt suicide. "Cutters" may want to stop cutting self but find stopping difficult, as this has become a *pattern of stress reduction.*

Groups at Risk for Suicide

- *Elderly* – especially those who are isolated, widowed; multiple losses, including friends/peers.
- *Males* – especially widowed and without close friends; sole emotional support came from marriage partner who is now deceased.
- *Adolescents and young adults.*
- *Serious/terminal illness* – not all terminally ill clients are suicidal, but should be considered in those who become depressed or hopeless.
- *Mood disorders* – depression and especially bipolar; always observe and assess those receiving treatment for depression, as suicide attempt may take place with improvement of depressive symptoms (client has the energy to commit suicide).
- *Schizophrenia* – newly diagnosed schizophrenics and those with command hallucinations.
- *Substance abusers* – especially with a mental disorder.
- *Stress and loss* – stressful situations and loss can trigger a suicide attempt, especially multiple stressors and losses or a significant loss.

Suicide Interventions

- Effective assessment and knowledge of risk factors
- Observation and safe environment (no "sharps")
- Psychopharmacology, especially the selected serotonin reuptake inhibitors (SSRIs) (children, adolescents, and young adults on SSRIs need to be closely monitored)
- Identification of triggers; educating client as to triggers to seek help early on
- Substance abuse treatment; treatment of pain disorders
- Psychotherapy/cognitive behavioral therapy/electroconvulsive therapy
- Treatment of medical disorders (thyroid/cancer)
- Increased activity if able
- Support network/family involvement
- Involvement in outside activities/avoid isolation – join outside groups, bereavement groups, organizations, care for a pet
- Client and family education

Elder Suicide (see Geriatric tab)

Terrorism/Disasters

With the increase in worldwide terrorism and natural disasters, health-care professionals need to improve their knowledge and awareness of the effects of psychological damage on individuals and communities affected by these disasters. In large-scale disasters:

- loss can involve individual homes/lives as well as whole communities (neighborhoods).
- neighbors and friends may be lost as well as reliable and familiar places and supports (neighborhoods, towns, rescue services).

Terrorism and War

- Loss may involve body parts (self-image) and a sense of trust and safety. Previous beliefs may be challenged.
- Individuals may experience shock, disorientation, anger, withdrawal, to name a few feelings/responses.
- The long-term effects on both individuals and future generations cannot be underestimated, and all health-care professionals need to familiarize themselves with disaster and terrorism preparedness.

Recent Wars/IEDs and PTSD

- In recent wars the use of IEDs and improved immediate medical care has resulted in soldiers surviving and then returning with traumatic brain injuries and the loss of multiple body parts.
- Homelessness has also increased for both men and women soldiers returning home, along with long separations of family members (mothers, fathers,

children), resulting in marital/family stress, and repeat tours of duty for men and women with little or no respite in between.

- Posttraumatic stress has "tripled," since 2001, among military personnel, who are combat exposed (Science News 2008). (See *Posttraumatic Stress Disorder* and *Substance-Related Disorders* in the Disorders-Interventions tab; see also *Smartphone Apps, PTSD Coach,* in Tools tab.)

Death and Dying/Grief

Stages of Death and Dying (Kübler-Ross)

1. *Denial and isolation* – usually temporary state of being unable to accept the possibility of one's death or that of a loved one.
2. *Anger* – replacement of temporary "stage one" with the reality that death is possible/going to happen. This is the realization that the future (plans/hopes) will have an end; a realization of the finality of the self. May fight/argue with health-care workers/push family/friends away.
3. *Bargaining* – seeks one last hope or possibility; enters an agreement or pact with God for "one last time or event" to take place before death. *(Let me live to see my grandchild born or my child graduate from college.)*
4. *Depression* – after time, loss, pain, the person realizes that the situation and course of illness will not improve; necessary stage to reach acceptance.
5. *Acceptance* – after working/passing through the previous stages, the person finally accepts what is going to happen; this is not resignation (giving up) or denying and fighting to the very end: it is a stage that allows for peace and dignity (Kübler-Ross 1997).

Complicated Versus Uncomplicated Grief

Complicated Grief	Uncomplicated Grief
• Excessive in duration (may be delayed reaction or compounded by losses [multiple losses]); usually longer than 3–6 mo • Disabling symptoms, morbid preoccupation with deceased/physical symptoms • Substance abuse, increased alcohol intake • Risk factors: limbo states (missing person), ambivalent relationship, multiple losses; long-term partner (sole dependency); no social network; history of depression • Suicidal thoughts–may want to join the deceased	• Follows a major loss • Depression perceived as normal • Self-esteem intact • Guilt specific to lost one (should have telephoned more) • Distress usually resolves within 12 wk (though mourning can continue for 1 or more years) • Suicidal thoughts transient or unusual (Shader 2003)

Victims of Abuse

Cycle of Battering

Phase I. Tension Building – Anger with little provocation; minor battering and excuses. Tension mounts and victim tries to placate. (Victim assumes guilt: I deserve to be abused.)

Phase II. Acute Battering – Most violent, up to 24 hours. Beating may be severe, and victim may provoke to get it over. Minimized by abuser. Help sought by victim if life-threatening or fear for children.

Phase III. Calm, Loving, Respite – Batterer is loving, kind, contrite. Fear of victim leaving. Lesson taught, and now batterer believes victim "understands."

- Victim believes batterer can change, and batterer uses guilt. Victim believes this (calm/loving in phase III) is *what batterer is really like.* Victim hopes the previous phases will not repeat themselves.
- Victim stays because of fear for life (batterer threatens more, and self-esteem lowers), society values marriage, divorce is viewed negatively, financial dependence.

Starts all over again – dangerous, and victim often killed (Walker 1979). Be aware that victims (of batterers) can be wives, husbands, intimate partners (female/female, male/male, male/female), and pregnant women.

Safety Plan (to Escape Abuser)

- Doors, windows, elevators – *rehearse exit plan.*
- *Have a place to go* – friends, relatives, motel – where you will be and feel safe.
- *Survival kit* – pack and *include money* (cab); change of clothes; identifying info (passports, birth certificate); legal documents, including protection orders; address books; jewelry; important papers.
- Start an *individual checking/savings account.*
- *Always have a safe exit* – do not argue in areas with no exit.
- *Legal rights/domestic hotlines* – know how to contact abuse/legal/domestic hotlines (see Web sites).
- *Review safety plan consistently* (monthly) (Reno 2004).

Signs of Child Abuse (Physical/Sexual)

Physical Abuse	Sexual Abuse
• Pattern of bruises/welts • Burns (e.g., from cigarettes, scalds) • Lesions resembling bites or fingernail marks • Unexplained fractures or dislocations, especially in child younger than 3 y • Areas of baldness from hair pulling • Injuries in various stages of healing • Other injuries or untreated illness, unrelated to present injury • X-rays revealing old fractures	• Signs of genital irritation, such as pain or itching • Bruised or bleeding genitalia • Enlarged vaginal or rectal orifice • Stains and/or blood on underwear • Unusual sexual behavior
Signs Common to Both	
• Signs of "failure to thrive" syndrome • Details of injury changing from person to person • History inconsistent with developmental stages • Parent blaming child or sibling for injury • Parental anger toward child for injury • Parental hostility toward health-care workers	• Exaggeration or absence of emotional response from parent regarding child's injury • Parent not providing child with comfort • Toddler or preschooler not protesting parent's leaving • Child showing preference for health-care worker over parent

Adapted from Myers RNotes 3rd ed., 2010, with permission.

Child Abuser Characteristics

Characteristics associated with those who may be child abusers:

- In a stressful situation, such as unemployed
- Poor coping strategies; may be suspicious or lose temper easily
- Isolated; few support systems or none
- Do not understand needs of children, basic care, or child development
- Expect child perfection, and child behavior blown out of proportion (Murray & Zentner 1997)

Incest

Often a father-daughter relationship (biological/stepfather), but can be father-son as well as mother-son.

- Child is made to feel special *(It is our special secret)*; gifts given.
- Favoritism (becomes intimate friend/sex partner replacing mother/other parent).

- Serious boundary violations and no safe place for child (child's bedroom usually used).
- May be threats if child tells about the sexual activities (Christianson & Blake 1990).

Signs of Incest

- Low self-esteem, sexual acting out, mood changes, sudden poor performance in school
- Parent spends inordinate amount of time with child, especially in room or late at night; very attentive to child
- Child is apprehensive (fearing sexual act/retaliation)
- Alcohol and drugs may be used (Christianson & Blake 1990)

ALERT: All child abuse (physical/sexual/emotional) or child neglect must be reported.

Elder Abuse (see Geriatric Tab)

Other Kinds of Abuse

- **Emotional Neglect** – parental/caretaker behaviors include:
  - Ignoring child
  - Ignoring needs (social, educational, developmental)
  - Rebuffing child's attempts at establishing interactions that are meaningful

  Little to no positive reinforcement (KCAPC 1992)
- **Emotional Injury** – results in serious impairment in child's functioning on all levels:
  - Treatment of child is harsh, with cruel and negative comments, belittling child
  - Child may behave immaturely, with inappropriate behaviors for age
  - Child demonstrates anxiety, fearfulness, sleep disturbances
  - Child shows inappropriate affect, self-destructive behaviors
  - Child may isolate, steal, cheat, as indication of emotional injury (KCAPC 1992)
- **Male Sexual Abuse** – Males are also sexually abused by mothers, fathers, uncles, pedophiles, and others in authority (coach, teacher, minister, priest)
  - Suffer from depression, shame, blame, guilt, and other effects of child sexual abuse
  - Issues related to masculinity, isolation, and struggles with seeking or receiving help
- **Worldwide Child Trafficking** – There are between 12 and 27 million people enslaved in the world today. Fifty percent are women and children and 1.2 million children are trafficked for child labor. An estimated 2 million children are trapped in sexual slavery around the world (www.worldvision.org 2010).
- **Child Pornography** – One of the fastest growing groups in the criminal justice system, likely fueled by Internet access (Hernandez 2009).

Geriatric/Elderly

Geriatric Assessment

Key Points

- Be mindful that the elderly client may be hard of hearing, but do not assume that all elderly are hard of hearing.
- Approach and speak to elderly clients as you would any other adult client. It is insulting to speak to the elderly client as if he/she were a child.
- Eye contact helps instill confidence and, in the presence of impaired hearing, will help the client to better understand you.
- Be aware that both decreased tactile sensation and ROM are normal changes with aging. Care should be taken to avoid unnecessary discomfort or even injury during a physical exam/assessment.
- Be aware of generational differences, especially gender differences (i.e., modesty for women, independence for men).
- Assess for altered mental states.
  - **Dementia:** Cognitive deficits (memory, reasoning, judgment, etc.)
  - **Delirium:** Confusion/excitement marked by disorientation to time and place, usually accompanied by illusions and/or hallucinations
  - **Depression:** Diminished interest or pleasure in most/all activities

Age-Related Changes and Their Implications

Decreased skin thickness	Elderly clients are more prone to skin breakdown
Decreased skin vascularity	Altered thermoregulation response can put elderly at risk for heatstroke

Continued

Age-Related Changes and Their Implications—cont'd

Loss of subcutaneous tissue	Decreased insulation can put elderly at risk for hypothermia
Decreased aortic elasticity	Produces increased diastolic blood pressure
Calcification of thoracic wall	Obscures heart and lung sounds and displaces apical pulse
Loss of nerve fibers/neurons	The elderly client needs extra time to learn and comprehend and to perform certain tasks
Decreased nerve conduction	Response to pain is altered
Reduced tactile sensation	Puts client at risk for accidental self-injury

From Myers, RNotes, 3rd ed., 2010, with permission

Disorders of Late Life

- **Dementia** – Dementia of the Alzheimer's type (AD), dementia with Lewy bodies, vascular and other dementias, delirium, and amnestic disorder *(see Delirium, Dementia, and Amnestic Disorders in the Disorders-Interventions tab).*
- **Geriatric depression** – Depression in old age is often assumed to be normal; however, depression at any age is not normal and needs to be diagnosed and treated. Factors can include:
  - Physical and cognitive decline
  - Loss of function/self-sufficiency
  - Loss of marriage partner, friends (narrowing support group), isolation
  - The elderly may have many somatic complaints (head hurts, stomach upsets) that mask the depression (Chenitz 1991) *(see Geriatric Depression Scale in Assessment tab)*
- **Pseudodementia** – Cognitive difficulty that is *actually caused by depression but may be mistaken for dementia.*
  - Need to consider and rule out dementia (Mini-Mental State Examination) and actually differentiate from depression (Geriatric Depression Scale)
  - Can be depressed with cognitive deficits as well
- **Late-onset schizophrenia** – Presents later in life, after age 60 y.
  - Psychotic episodes (delusions or hallucinations) may be overlooked (schizophrenia is considered to be a young-adult disease)
  - Organic brain disease should be considered as part of the differential diagnosis

Characteristics of Late-Onset Schizophrenia

- *Delusions of persecution* common, hallucinations prominent; "partition" delusion (people/objects pass through barriers and enter home) common; rare in early onset.
- *Sensory deficits* – often auditory/visual impairments
- May have been *previously paranoid, reclusive,* yet functioned otherwise
- *Lives alone/isolated/unmarried*
- *Negative symptoms/thought disorder rare*
- *More common in women* (early onset: equally common) (Lubman & Castle 2002)

Psychotropic Drugs – Geriatric Considerations

(See Drugs A–Z tab for geriatric considerations; and the Elderly and Medications [Drugs/Labs tab].)

Pharmacokinetics in the Elderly

Pharmacokinetics is the way that a drug is absorbed, distributed and used, metabolized, and excreted by the body. Age-related physiological changes affect body systems, altering pharmacokinetics and increasing or altering a drug's effect.

Physiological	Effect on Change	Pharmacokinetics
Absorption	• Decreased intestinal motility	Delayed peak effect
	• Diminished blood flow to the gut	Delayed signs/symptoms of toxic effects
Distribution	• Decreased body water	Increased serum concentration of water-soluble drugs
	• Increased percentage of body fat	Increased half-life of fat-soluble drugs
	• Decreased amount of plasma proteins	Increased amount of active drug
	• Decreased lean body mass	Increased drug concentration
Metabolism	• Decreased blood flow to liver	Decreased rate of drug clearance by liver
	• Diminished liver function	Increased accumulation of some drugs

Continued

Physiological	Effect on Change	Pharmacokinetics
Excretion	• Diminished kidney function	Increased accumulation of drugs excreted by kidney
	• Decreased creatinine clearance	

From Myers, RNotes, 3rd ed., 2010, with permission

Elder Abuse

There are many types of elder abuse, which include:

- *Elder neglect* (lack of care by omission or commission)
- *Psychological* or *emotional abuse* (verbal assaults, insults, threats)
- *Physical* (physical injury, pain, drugs, restraints)
- *Sexual abuse* (nonconsensual sex: rape, sodomy)
- *Financial abuse* (misuse of resources: social security, property)
- *Self-neglect* (elder cannot provide appropriate self care)

Elder Abuse – Physical Signs

- Hematomas, welts, bites, burns, bruises, and pressure sores
- Fractures (various stages of healing), contractures
- Rashes, fecal impaction
- Weight loss, dehydration, substandard personal hygiene
- Broken dentures, hearing aids, other devices; poor oral hygiene; traumatic alopecia; subconjunctival hemorrhage

Elder Abuse – Behavioral Signs

Caregiver

- Caregiver insistence on being present during entire appointment
- Answers for client
- Caregiver expresses indifference or anger, not offering assistance
- Caregiver does not visit hospitalized client

Elder

- Hesitation to be open, appearing fearful, poor eye contact, ashamed, baby talk
- Paranoia, anxiety, anger, low self-esteem
- *Physical signs:* contractures, inconsistent medication regimen (subtherapeutic levels), malnutrition, poor hygiene, dehydration
- *Financial:* signed over power of attorney (unwillingly), possessions gone, lack of money

Elder Abuse – Medical and Psychiatric History

- Mental health/psychiatric interview
- Assess for depression, anxiety, alcohol (substance) abuse, insomnia
- Functional independence/dependence
- Cognitive impairment (Stiles et al 2002)

◎ **ALERT:** All elder abuse must be reported.

Elder Suicide

Warning Signs

- Failed suicide attempt
- *Indirect clues* – stockpiling medications; purchasing a gun; putting affairs in order; making/changing a will; donating body to science; giving possessions/money away; relationship, social downturns; recent appointment with a physician
- *Situational clues* – recent move, death of spouse/friend/child
- *Symptoms* – depression, insomnia, agitation, others

Elder Profile for Potential Suicide

- Male gender
- White
- Divorced or widowed
- Lives alone, isolated, moved recently
- Unemployed, retired
- Poor health, pain, multiple illnesses, terminal
- Depressed, substance abuser, hopeless
- Family history of suicide, depression, substance abuse; harsh parenting, early trauma in childhood
- Wish to end hopeless, intolerable situation
- *Lethal means:* guns, stockpiled sedatives/hypnotics
- Previous attempt
- Not inclined to reach out; often somatic complaints

Suspected Elder Suicidality

Ask direct questions:

- *Are you so down you see no point in going on?* (If answer is yes, explore further: *Tell me more.*)
- *Have you (ever) thought of killing yourself? (When? What stopped you?)*
- *How often do you have these thoughts?*
- *How would you kill yourself?* (Lethality plan) (Holkup 2002)

Gather information – keep communication open in a nonjudgmental way; do not minimize or offer advice in this situation.

Tools/References/Index

The following are located on DavisPlus (PsychNotes) at: http://davisplus.fadavis.com

- Psychotropic Drugs (over 75 complete monographs)
- Psychiatric Assessment Rating Scale Information
- Psychiatric Resources: Organizations/Web sites/Hotlines

Abbreviations

AD Dementia of Alzheimer's type
ADHD Attention deficit hyperactivity disorder
AE Adverse event
AIMS Abnormal Involuntary Movement Scale
BAI Beck Anxiety Inventory
BDI Beck Depression Inventory
BP Blood pressure
BPD Borderline personality disorder
BPH Benign prostatic hypertrophy
CBC Complete blood count
CBT Cognitive behavioral therapy
CHF Congestive heart failure
CK Creatine kinase
CNS Central nervous system
COPD Chronic obstructive pulmonary disease
CT scan Computed tomography scan
CV Cardiovascular
DBT Dialectical behavioral therapy
d/c Discontinue
ECA Epidemiologic Catchment Area Survey
ECG Electrocardiogram
ECT Electroconvulsive therapy
EMDR Eye movement desensitization and reprocessing
EPS Extrapyramidal symptoms
FBS Fasting blood sugar
GABA Gamma-aminobutyric acid
GAD Generalized anxiety disorder
GDS Geriatric Depression Scale
Hx History
LFTs Liver function tests
IM Intramuscular
IV Intravenous
kg Kilogram
L Liter
MAOI Monoamine oxidase inhibitor
MCV Mean corpuscular volume
MDD Major depressive disorder
μg Microgram
mEq Milliequivalent
MH Mental health
mL Milliliter
MMSE Mini-Mental State Exam
MRI Magnetic resonance imaging
MSE Mental Status Exam
NAMI National Association for the Mentally Ill
NE Norepinephrine
NMS Neuroleptic malignant syndrome
OCD Obsessive-compulsive disorder
OTC Over the counter
PANSS Positive and Negative Syndrome Scale
PMDD Premenstrual dysphoric disorder
PTSD Posttraumatic stress disorder
SMAST Short Michigan Alcohol Screening Test
SNRI Serotonin-norepinephrine reuptake inhibitor
SSRI Selective serotonin reuptake inhibitor
$T_{1/2}$ Drug's half-life
TCA Tricyclic antidepressant
TFT Thyroid function test
TIA Transient ischemic attack
TPR Temperature, pulse, respiration
UA Urinalysis
UTI Urinary tract infection

Assessment Tools

See Assessment Tab for the following tools/rating scales:

- Abnormal Involuntary Movement Scale (AIMS)
- Depression-Arkansas Scale (D-ARK scale)
- DSM-IV Multiaxial Assessment Tool
- Edinburgh Postnatal Depression Scale (EPDS)
- Geriatric Depression Scale (GDS)
- Global Assessment of Functioning (GAF) Scale
- Ethnocultural Assessment Tool
- Mental Status Assessment Tool
- Mood Disorder Questionnaire (MDQ)
- Psychiatric History and Assessment Tool
- Short Michigan Alcohol Screening Test (SMAST)
- Substance History and Assessment

Smartphone Apps

An increasing number of self-rating mood disorder apps are being developed for smartphones for consumer use. Disclaimers state, rightfully so, that these tools are "for information purposes only" or "not to be used as a diagnostic tool." As long as the consumer understands the tool is not providing an actual diagnosis and seeks professional help when a red flag is raised, the screening may have provided a service. However, without validation of the screening tool, caution is advised and professional evaluation should be advised.

Validated App & Mood/Anxiety Disorder Screening Tool: MYM3 – My Mood Monitor (M-3 Checklist)

The M-3 Checklist was developed by a team of psychiatrists, family physicians, psychologists, and others and validated in a study performed at the University of North Carolina (Gaynes 2010).

- Three-minute, 27-item rating scale that screens for mood and anxiety disorders, including depression, anxiety, PTSD, and Bipolar that can be used in primary care.
- Mym3 app for smartphone costs about $2.99.
- Diagnostic accuracy equals current single-disorder screens.
- If there is a red flag for suicide, user can immediately call the National Suicide Prevention Hotline.
- M-3 score of 33 or higher suggests a mood disorder and degree of severity is provided for all four categories, e.g., low, medium, high.
- User can monitor progress (graphically) and treatments at: mymoodmonitor.com

Other Apps

- **PTSD Coach** – A free educational, self-assessment, and symptom management app for veterans and others with PTSD, though military oriented (Department of Veterans Affairs 2011; http://ptsd.va.gov/).
- **Additional Apps include**: Sad Scale (four depression scales), Depression Test and Self Tracker (Goldberg Scale). Likely more apps will be developed and others replaced, but mental health professionals should be aware of their existence (and use by consumers) and use caution with apps that do not use validated screening tools.

DSM-IV-TR Classification: Axes I and II Categories and Codes

Disorders Usually First Diagnosed In Infancy, Childhood, or Adolescence

Mental Retardation

NOTE: *These are coded on Axis II.*

317 Mild Mental Retardation
318.0 Moderate Retardation
318.1 Severe Retardation
318.2 Profound Mental Retardation
319 Mental Retardation, Severity Unspecified

Learning Disorders

315.00 Reading Disorder
315.1 Mathematics Disorder
315.2 Disorder of Written Expression
315.9 Learning Disorder Not Otherwise Specified (NOS)

Motor Skills Disorder

315.4 Developmental Coordination Disorder

Communication Disorders

315.31 Expressive Language Disorder
315.32 Mixed Receptive-Expressive Language Disorder
315.39 Phonological Disorder
307.0 Stuttering
307.9 Communication Disorder NOS

Pervasive Developmental Disorders

299.00 Autistic Disorder
299.80 Rett's Disorder
299.10 Childhood Disintegrative Disorder
299.80 Asperger's Disorder
299.80 Pervasive Developmental Disorder NOS

Attention-Deficit and Disruptive Behavior Disorders
314.xx Attention-Deficit/Hyperactivity Disorder
314.01 Combined Type
314.00 Predominantly Inattentive Type
314.01 Predominantly Hyperactive-Impulsive Type
314.9 Attention-Deficit/Hyperactivity Disorder NOS
312.xx Conduct Disorder
.81 Childhood-Onset Type
.82 Adolescent-Onset Type
.89 Unspecified Onset
313.81 Oppositional Defiant Disorder
312.9 Disruptive Behavior Disorder NOS

Feeding and Eating Disorders of Infancy or Early Childhood
307.52 Pica
307.53 Rumination Disorder
307.59 Feeding Disorder of Infancy or Early Childhood

Tic Disorders
307.23 Tourette's Disorder
307.22 Chronic Motor or Vocal Tic Disorder
307.21 Transient Tic Disorder
307.20 Tic Disorder NOS

Elimination Disorders
—.– Encopresis
787.6 With Constipation and Overflow Incontinence
307.7 Without Constipation and Overflow Incontinence
307.6 Enuresis (Not Due to a General Medical Condition)

Other Disorders of Infancy, Childhood, or Adolescence
309.21 Separation Anxiety Disorder
313.23 Selective Mutism
313.89 Reactive Attachment Disorder of Infancy or Early Childhood
307.3 Stereotypic Movement Disorder
313.9 Disorder of Infancy, Childhood, or Adolescence NOS

Delirium, Dementia, and Amnestic and Other Cognitive Disorders

Delirium
293.0 Delirium Due to ... *(Indicate the general medical condition)*
—.– Substance Intoxication Delirium *(refer to Substance-Related Disorders for substance-specific codes)*
—.– Substance Withdrawal Delirium *(refer to Substance-Related Disorders for substance-specific codes)*

——.— Delirium Due to Multiple Etiologies *(code each of the specific etiologies)*
780.09 Delirium NOS

Dementia

294.xx* Dementia of the Alzheimer's Type, With Early Onset
.10 Without Behavioral Disturbance
.11 With Behavioral Disturbance
294.xx* Dementia of the Alzheimer's Type, With Late Onset
.10 Without Behavioral Disturbance
.11 With Behavioral Disturbance
290.xx Vascular Dementia
.40 Uncomplicated
.41 With Delirium
.42 With Delusions
.43 With Depressed Mood
294.1x* Dementia Due to HIV Disease
294.1x* Dementia Due to Head Trauma
294.1x* Dementia Due to Parkinson's Disease
294.1x* Dementia Due to Huntington's Disease
294.1x* Dementia Due to Pick's Disease
294.1x* Dementia Due to Creutzfeldt-Jakob Disease
294.1x* Dementia Due to *(indicate the general medical condition not listed above)*
——.— Substance-Induced Persisting Dementia *(refer to Substance-Related Disorders for substance-specific codes)*
——.— Dementia Due to Multiple Etiologies (code each of the specific etiologies)
294.8 Dementia NOS

---

*Also add ICD–9–CM codes valid after October 1, 2000 on Axis III for these disorders.

Amnestic Disorders

294.0 Amnestic Disorder Due to *(indicate the general medical condition)*
——.— Substance-Induced Persisting Amnestic Disorder *(refer to Substance-Related Disorders for substance-specific codes)*
294.8 Amnestic Disorder NOS

Other Cognitive Disorders

294.9 Cognitive Disorder NOS

Mental Disorders Due to a General Medical Condition Not Elsewhere Classified

293.89 Catatonic Disorder Due to *(indicate the general medical condition)*
310.1 Personality Change Due to *(indicate the general medical condition)*
293.9 Mental Disorder NOS Due to *(indicate the general medical condition)*

Substance-Related Disorders

Alcohol-Related Disorders

Alcohol Use Disorders

303.90 Alcohol Dependence
305.00 Alcohol Abuse

Alcohol-Induced Disorders

303.00 Alcohol Intoxication
291.81 Alcohol Withdrawal
291.0 Alcohol Intoxication Delirium
291.0 Alcohol Withdrawal Delirium
291.2 Alcohol-Induced Persisting Dementia
291.1 Alcohol-Induced Persisting Amnestic Disorder
291.x Alcohol-Induced Psychotic Disorder
  .5 With Delusions
  .3 With Hallucinations
291.89 Alcohol-Induced Mood Disorder
291.89 Alcohol-Induced Anxiety Disorder
291.89 Alcohol-Induced Sexual Dysfunction
291.89 Alcohol-Induced Sleep Disorder
291.9 Alcohol-Related Disorder NOS

Amphetamine (or Amphetamine-like)-Related Disorders

Amphetamine Use Disorders

304.40 Amphetamine Dependence
305.70 Amphetamine Abuse

Amphetamine-Induced Disorders

292.89 Amphetamine Intoxication
292.0 Amphetamine Withdrawal
292.81 Amphetamine Intoxication Delirium
292.xx Amphetamine-Induced Psychotic Disorder
  .11 With Delusions
  .12 With Hallucinations
292.84 Amphetamine-Induced Mood Disorder
292.89 Amphetamine-Induced Anxiety Disorder
292.89 Amphetamine-Induced Sexual Dysfunction
292.89 Amphetamine-Induced Sleep Disorder
292.9 Amphetamine-Related Disorder NOS

Caffeine-Related Disorders

Caffeine-Induced Disorders

305.90 Caffeine Intoxication
292.89 Caffeine-Induced Anxiety Disorder

292.89 Caffeine-Induced Sleep Disorder
292.9 Caffeine-Related Disorder NOS

Cannabis-Related Disorders

Cannabis Use Disorders

304.30 Cannabis Dependence
305.20 Cannabis Abuse

Cannabis-Induced Disorders

292.89 Cannabis Intoxication
292.81 Cannabis Intoxication Delirium
292.xx Cannabis-Induced Psychotic Disorder
.11 With Delusions
.12 With Hallucinations
292.89 Cannabis-Induced Anxiety Disorder
292.9 Cannabis-Related Disorder NOS

Cocaine-Related Disorders

Cocaine Use Disorders

304.20 Cocaine Dependence
305.60 Cocaine Abuse

Cocaine-Induced Disorders

292.89 Cocaine Intoxication
292.0 Cocaine Withdrawal
292.81 Cocaine Intoxication Delirium
292.xx Cocaine-Induced Psychotic Disorder
.11 With Delusions
.12 With Hallucinations
292.84 Cocaine-Induced Mood Disorder
292.89 Cocaine-Induced Anxiety Disorder
292.89 Cocaine-Induced Sexual Dysfunction
292.89 Cocaine-Induced Sleep Disorder
292.9 Cocaine-Related Disorder NOS

Hallucinogen-Related Disorders

Hallucinogen Use Disorders

304.50 Hallucinogen Dependence
305.30 Hallucinogen Abuse

Hallucinogen-Induced Disorders

292.89 Hallucinogen Intoxication
292.89 Hallucinogen Persisting Perception Disorder (Flashbacks)
292.81 Hallucinogen Intoxication Delirium
292.xx Hallucinogen-Induced Psychotic Disorder

.11 With Delusions
.12 With Hallucinations
292.84 Hallucinogen-Induced Mood Disorder
292.89 Hallucinogen-Induced Anxiety Disorder
292.9 Hallucinogen-Related Disorder NOS

Inhalant-Related Disorders

Inhalant Use Disorders

304.60 Inhalant Dependence
305.90 Inhalant Abuse

Inhalant-Induced Disorders

292.89 Inhalant Intoxication
292.81 Inhalant Intoxication Delirium
292.82 Inhalant-Induced Persisting Dementia
292.xx Inhalant-Induced Psychotic Disorder
.11 With Delusions
.12 With Hallucinations
292.84 Inhalant-Induced Mood Disorder
292.89 Inhalant-Induced Anxiety Disorder
292.9 Inhalant-Related Disorder NOS

Nicotine-Related Disorders

Nicotine Use Disorders

305.1 Nicotine Dependence

Nicotine-Induced Disorders

292.0 Nicotine Withdrawal
292.9 Nicotine-Related Disorder NOS

Opioid-Related Disorders

Opioid Use Disorders

304.00 Opioid Dependence
305.50 Opioid Abuse

Opioid-Induced Disorders

292.89 Opioid Intoxication
292.0 Opioid Withdrawal
292.81 Opioid Intoxication Delirium
292.xx Opioid-Induced Psychotic Disorder
.11 With Delusions
.12 With Hallucinations
292.84 Opioid-Induced Mood Disorder
292.89 Opioid-Induced Sexual Dysfunction
292.89 Opioid-Induced Sleep Disorder
292.9 Opioid-Related Disorder NOS

Phencyclidine (or Phencyclidine-like)-Related Disorders

Phencyclidine Use Disorders

304.60 Phencyclidine Dependence
305.90 Phencyclidine Abuse

Phencyclidine-Induced Disorders

292.89 Phencyclidine Intoxication
292.81 Phencyclidine Intoxication Delirium
292.xx Phencyclidine-Induced Psychotic Disorder
    .11 With Delusions
    .12 With Hallucinations
292.84 Phencyclidine-Induced Mood Disorder
292.89 Phencyclidine-Induced Anxiety Disorder
292.9 Phencyclidine-Related Disorder NOS

Sedative-, Hypnotic-, or Anxiolytic-Related Disorders

Sedative, Hypnotic, or Anxiolytic Use Disorders

304.10 Sedative, Hypnotic, or Anxiolytic Dependence
305.40 Sedative, Hypnotic, or Anxiolytic Abuse

Sedative-, Hypnotic-, or Anxiolytic-Induced Disorders

292.89 Sedative, Hypnotic, or Anxiolytic Intoxication
292.0 Sedative, Hypnotic, or Anxiolytic Withdrawal
292.81 Sedative, Hypnotic, or Anxiolytic Intoxication Delirium
292.81 Sedative, Hypnotic, or Anxiolytic Withdrawal Delirium
292.82 Sedative-, Hypnotic-, or Anxiolytic-Induced Persisting Dementia
292.83 Sedative-, Hypnotic-, or Anxiolytic-Induced Persisting Amnestic Disorder
292.xx Sedative-, Hypnotic-, or Anxiolytic-Induced Psychotic Disorder
    .11 With Delusions
    .12 With Hallucinations
292.84 Sedative-, Hypnotic-, or Anxiolytic-Induced Mood Disorder
292.89 Sedative-, Hypnotic-, or Anxiolytic-Induced Anxiety Disorder
292.89 Sedative-, Hypnotic-, or Anxiolytic-Induced Sexual Dysfunction
292.89 Sedative-, Hypnotic-, or Anxiolytic-Induced Sleep Disorder
292.9 Sedative-, Hypnotic-, or Anxiolytic-Related Disorder NOS

Polysubstance-Related Disorder

304.80 Polysubstance Dependence

Other (or Unknown) Substance-Related Disorders

Other (or Unknown) Substance Use Disorders

304.90 Other (or Unknown) Substance Dependence
305.90 Other (or Unknown) Substance Abuse

Other (or Unknown) Substance-Induced Disorders

292.89 Other (or Unknown) Substance Intoxication
292.0 Other (or Unknown) Substance Withdrawal
292.81 Other (or Unknown) Substance-Induced Delirium
292.82 Other (or Unknown) Substance-Induced Persisting Dementia
292.83 Other (or Unknown) Substance-Induced Persisting Amnestic Disorder
292.xx Other (or Unknown) Substance-Induced Psychotic Disorder
 .11 With Delusions
 .12 With Hallucinations
292.84 Other (or Unknown) Substance-Induced Mood Disorder
292.89 Other (or Unknown) Substance-Induced Anxiety Disorder
292.89 Other (or Unknown) Substance-Induced Sexual Dysfunction
292.89 Other (or Unknown) Substance-Induced Sleep Disorder
292.9 Other (or Unknown) Substance-Related Disorder NOS

Schizophrenia and Other Psychotic Disorders

295.xx Schizophrenia
 .30 Paranoid type
 .10 Disorganized type
 .20 Catatonic type
 .90 Undifferentiated type
 .60 Residual type
295.40 Schizophreniform Disorder
295.70 Schizoaffective Disorder
297.1 Delusional Disorder
298.8 Brief Psychotic Disorder
297.3 Shared Psychotic Disorder
293.xx Psychotic Disorder Due to *(indicate the general medical condition)*
 .81 With Delusions
 .82 With Hallucinations
—.— Substance-Induced Psychotic Disorder *(refer to Substance-Related Disorders for substance-specific codes)*
298.9 Psychotic Disorder NOS

Mood Disorders

(Code current state of Major Depressive Disorder or Bipolar I Disorder in fifth digit: 0 = unspecified; 1 = mild; 2 = moderate; 3 = severe, without psychotic features; 4 = severe, with psychotic features; 5 = in partial remission; 6 = in full remission)

Depressive Disorders

296.xx Major Depressive Disorder
 .2x Single Episode
 .3x Recurrent
300.4 Dysthymic Disorder
311 Depressive Disorder NOS

Bipolar Disorders

296.xx Bipolar I Disorder
- .0x Single Manic Episode
- .40 Most Recent Episode Hypomanic
- .4x Most Recent Episode Manic
- .6x Most Recent Episode Mixed
- .5x Most Recent Episode Depressed
- .7 Most Recent Episode Unspecified

296.89 Bipolar II Disorder *(specify current or most recent episode: Hypomanic or Depressed)*
301.13 Cyclothymic Disorder
296.80 Bipolar Disorder NOS
293.83 Mood Disorder Due to *(indicate the general medical condition)*
—.— Substance-Induced Mood Disorder *(refer to Substance-Related Disorders for substance-specific codes)*
296.90 Mood Disorder NOS

Anxiety Disorders

300.01 Panic Disorder Without Agoraphobia
300.21 Panic Disorder With Agoraphobia
300.22 Agoraphobia Without History of Panic Disorder
300.29 Specific Phobia
300.23 Social Phobia
300.3 Obsessive-Compulsive Disorder
309.81 Posttraumatic Stress Disorder
308.3 Acute Stress Disorder
300.02 Generalized Anxiety Disorder
293.89 Anxiety Disorder Due to *(indicate the general medical condition)*
—.— Substance-Induced Anxiety Disorder *(refer to Substance-Related Disorders for substance-specific codes)*
300.00 Anxiety Disorder NOS

Somatoform Disorders

300.81 Somatization Disorder
300.82 Undifferentiated Somatoform Disorder
300.11 Conversion Disorder
307.xx Pain Disorder
- .80 Associated with Psychological Factors
- .89 Associated with Both Psychological Factors and a General Medical Condition

300.7 Hypochondriasis
300.7 Body Dysmorphic Disorder
300.82 Somatoform Disorder NOS

Factitious Disorders

300.xx Factitious Disorder
  .16 With Predominantly Psychological Signs and Symptoms
  .19 With Predominantly Physical Signs and Symptoms
  .19 With Combined Psychological and Physical Signs and Symptoms
300.19 Factitious Disorder NOS

Dissociative Disorders

300.12 Dissociative Amnesia
300.13 Dissociative Fugue
300.14 Dissociative Identity Disorder
300.6 Depersonalization Disorder
300.15 Dissociative Disorder NOS

Sexual and Gender Identity Disorders

Sexual Dysfunctions

Sexual Desire Disorders

302.71 Hypoactive Sexual Desire Disorder
302.79 Sexual Aversion Disorder

Sexual Arousal Disorders

302.72 Female Sexual Arousal Disorder
302.72 Male Erectile Disorder

Orgasmic Disorders

302.73 Female Orgasmic Disorder
302.74 Male Orgasmic Disorder
302.75 Premature Ejaculation

Sexual Pain Disorders

302.76 Dyspareunia (Not Due to a General Medical Condition)
306.51 Vaginismus (Not Due to a General Medical Condition)

Sexual Dysfunction Due to a General Medical Condition

625.8 Female Hypoactive Sexual Desire Disorder Due to *(indicate the general medical condition)*
608.89 Male Hypoactive Sexual Desire Disorder Due to *(indicate the general medical condition)*
607.84 Male Erectile Disorder Due to *(indicate the general medical condition)*
625.0 Female Dyspareunia Due to *(indicate the general medical condition)*
608.89 Male Dyspareunia Due to *(indicate the general medical condition)*
625.8 Other Female Sexual Dysfunction Due to *(indicate the general medical condition)*
608.89 Other Male Sexual Dysfunction Due to *(indicate the general medical condition)*

—— .— Substance-Induced Sexual Dysfunction *(refer to Substance-Related Disorders for substance-specific codes)*
302.70 Sexual Dysfunction NOS

Paraphilias
302.4 Exhibitionism
302.81 Fetishism
302.89 Frotteurism
302.2 Pedophilia
302.83 Sexual Masochism
302.84 Sexual Sadism
302.3 Transvestic Fetishism
302.82 Voyeurism
302.9 Paraphilia NOS

Gender Identity Disorders
302.xx Gender Identity Disorder
.6 In Children
.85 In Adolescents or Adults
302.6 Gender Identity Disorder NOS
302.9 Sexual Disorder NOS

Eating Disorders
307.1 Anorexia Nervosa
307.51 Bulimia Nervosa
307.50 Eating Disorder NOS

Sleep Disorders

Primary Sleep Disorders

Dyssomnias
307.42 Primary Insomnia
307.44 Primary Hypersomnia
347 Narcolepsy
780.59 Breathing-Related Sleep Disorder
307.45 Circadian Rhythm Sleep Disorder
307.47 Dyssomnia NOS

Parasomnias
307.47 Nightmare Disorder
307.46 Sleep Terror Disorder
307.46 Sleepwalking Disorder
307.47 Parasomnia NOS

Sleep Disorders Related to Another Mental Disorder
307.42 Insomnia Related to *(indicate the Axis I or Axis II disorder)*
307.44 Hypersomnia Related to *(indicate the Axis I or Axis II disorder)*

Other Sleep Disorders

780.xx Sleep Disorder Due to *(indicate the general medical condition)*
- .52 Insomnia type
- .54 Hypersomnia type
- .59 Parasomnia type
- .59 Mixed type

Substance-Induced Sleep Disorder *(refer to Substance-Related Disorders for substance-specific codes)*

Impulse Control Disorders Not Elsewhere Classified

312.34 Intermittent Explosive Disorder
312.32 Kleptomania
312.33 Pyromania
312.31 Pathological Gambling
312.39 Trichotillomania
312.30 Impulse Control Disorder NOS

Adjustment Disorders

309.xx Adjustment Disorder
- .0 With Depressed Mood
- .24 With Anxiety
- .28 With Mixed Anxiety and Depressed Mood
- .3 With Disturbance of Conduct
- .4 With Mixed Disturbance of Emotions and Conduct
- .9 Unspecified

Personality Disorders

NOTE: *These are coded on Axis II.*

301.0 Paranoid Personality Disorder
301.20 Schizoid Personality Disorder
301.22 Schizotypal Personality Disorder
301.7 Antisocial Personality Disorder
301.83 Borderline Personality Disorder
301.50 Histrionic Personality Disorder
301.81 Narcissistic Personality Disorder
301.82 Avoidant Personality Disorder
301.6 Dependent Personality Disorder
301.4 Obsessive-Compulsive Personality Disorder
301.9 Personality Disorder NOS

Other Conditions That May Be a Focus of Clinical Attention

Psychological Factors Affecting Medical Condition

316 *Choose name based on nature of factors:*
Mental Disorder Affecting Medical Condition

Psychological Symptoms Affecting Medical Condition
Personality Traits or Coping Style Affecting Medical Condition
Maladaptive Health Behaviors Affecting Medical Condition
Stress-Related Physiological Response Affecting Medical Condition
Other or Unspecified Psychological Factors Affecting Medical Condition

Medication-Induced Movement Disorders

332.1 Neuroleptic-Induced Parkinsonism
333.92 Neuroleptic Malignant Syndrome
333.7 Neuroleptic-Induced Acute Dystonia
333.99 Neuroleptic-Induced Acute Akathisia
333.82 Neuroleptic-Induced Tardive Dyskinesia
333.1 Medication-Induced Postural Tremor
333.90 Medication-Induced Movement Disorder NOS

Other Medication-Induced Disorder

995.2 Adverse Effects of Medication NOS

Relational Problems

V61.9 Relational Problem Related to a Mental Disorder or General Medical Condition
V61.20 Parent-Child Relational Problem
V61.10 Partner Relational Problem
V61.8 Sibling Relational Problem
V62.81 Relational Problem NOS

Problems Related to Abuse or Neglect

V61.21 Physical Abuse of Child
V61.21 Sexual Abuse of Child
V61.21 Neglect of Child
—.— Physical Abuse of Adult
V61.12 (if by partner)
V62.83 (if by person other than partner)
—.—Sexual Abuse of Adult
V61.12 (if by partner)
V62.83 (if by person other than partner)

Additional Conditions That May Be a Focus of Clinical Attention

V15.81 Noncompliance with Treatment
V65.2 Malingering
V71.01 Adult Antisocial Behavior
V71.02 Childhood or Adolescent Antisocial Behavior
V62.89 Borderline Intellectual Functioning (coded on Axis II)
780.9 Age-Related Cognitive Decline
V62.82 Bereavement

V62.3 Academic Problem
V62.2 Occupational Problem
313.82 Identity Problem
V62.89 Religious or Spiritual Problem
V62.4 Acculturation Problem
V62.89 Phase of Life Problem

Additional Codes

300.9 Unspecified Mental Disorder (nonpsychotic)
V71.09 No Diagnosis or Condition on Axis I
799.9 Diagnosis or Condition Deferred on Axis I
V71.09 No Diagnosis on Axis II
799.9 Diagnosis Deferred on Axis II

DSM-IV-TR criteria in Disorders Tab, Global Assessment of Functioning (GAF) form, Multiaxial System, and DSM-IV-TR classifications: Axes I and II categories and codes, reprinted with permission from the Diagnostic and Statistical Manual of Mental Disorders, 4th ed., Text Revision. Washington, DC: American Psychiatric Association, 2000.

Assigning Nursing Diagnoses (NANDA) to Client Behaviors

Following is a list of client behaviors and the NANDA nursing diagnoses that correspond to the behaviors and that may be used in planning care for the client exhibiting the specific behavioral symptoms.

Behaviors	NANDA Nursing Diagnoses
Aggression; hostility	Risk for injury; Risk for other-directed violence
Anorexia or refusal to eat	Imbalanced nutrition: Less than body requirements
Anxious behavior	Anxiety (specify level)
Confusion; memory loss	Confusion, acute/chronic; Disturbed thought processes
Delusions	Disturbed thought processes
Denial of problems	Ineffective denial
Depressed mood or anger turned inward	Dysfunctional grieving

Continued

Behaviors	NANDA Nursing Diagnoses
Detoxification; withdrawal from substances	Risk for injury
Difficulty making important life decision	Decisional conflict (specify)
Difficulty with interpersonal relationships	Impaired social interaction
Disruption in capability to perform usual responsibilities	Ineffective role performance
Dissociative behaviors (depersonalization; derealization)	Disturbed sensory perception (kinesthetic)
Expresses feelings of disgust about body or body part	Disturbed body image
Expresses lack of control over personal situation	Powerlessness
Flashbacks, nightmares, obsession with traumatic experience	Posttrauma syndrome
Hallucinations	Disturbed sensory perception (auditory; visual)
Highly critical of self or others	Low self-esteem (chronic; situational)
HIV-positive; altered immunity	Ineffective protection
Inability to meet basic needs	Self-care deficit (feeding; bathing/ hygiene; dressing/grooming; toileting)
Insomnia or hypersomnia	Disturbed sleep pattern
Loose associations or flight of ideas	Impaired verbal communication
Manic hyperactivity	Risk for injury
Manipulative behavior	Ineffective coping
Multiple personalities; gender identity disturbance	Disturbed personal identity
Orgasm, problems with; lack of sexual desire	Sexual dysfunction
Overeating, compulsive	Risk for imbalanced nutrition: More than body requirements
Phobias	Fear
Physical symptoms as coping behavior	Ineffective coping

Continued

Behaviors	NANDA Nursing Diagnoses
Projection of blame; rationalization of failures; denial of personal responsibility	Defensive coping
Ritualistic behaviors	Anxiety (severe); Ineffective coping
Seductive remarks; inappropriate sexual behaviors	Impaired social interaction
Self-mutilative behaviors	Self-mutilation; Risk for self-mutilation
Sexual behaviors (difficulty, limitations, or changes in; reported dissatisfaction)	Ineffective sexuality patterns
Stress from caring for chronically ill person	Caregiver role strain
Stress from locating to new environment	Relocation stress syndrome
Substance use as a coping behavior	Ineffective coping
Substance use (denies use is a problem)	Ineffective denial
Suicidal	Risk for suicide; Risk for self-directed violence
Suspiciousness	Disturbed thought processes; Ineffective coping
Vomiting, excessive, self induced	Risk for deficient fluid volume
Withdrawn behavior	Social isolation

Used with permission from Townsend, 5e 2010

Nursing Diagnoses (NANDA) (2009–2011)

Access NANDA by Doenges and Moorehouse Diagnostic Division online at Davis's Nursing Resource Center at: http://davisplus.fadavis.com/daviscareplans/index.cfm

Psychiatric Terminology

A

abreaction. "Remembering with feeling"; bringing into conscious awareness painful events that have been repressed and reexperiencing the emotions that were associated with the events.

adjustment disorder. A maladaptive reaction to an identifiable psychosocial stressor that occurs within 3 months after onset of the stressor. The individual shows impairment in social and occupational functioning or exhibits symptoms that are in excess of a normal and expectable reaction to the stressor.

affect. The behavioral expression of emotion; may be appropriate (congruent with the situation); inappropriate (incongruent with the situation); constricted or blunted (diminished range and intensity); or flat (absence of emotional expression).

agoraphobia. The fear of being in places or situations from which escape might be difficult (or embarrassing) or in which help might not be available in the event of a panic attack.

akathisia. Restlessness; an urgent need for movement. A type of extrapyramidal side effect associated with some antipsychotic medications.

akinesia. Muscular weakness or a loss or partial loss of muscle movement; a type of extrapyramidal side effect associated with some antipsychotic medications.

amnesia. An inability to recall important personal information that is too extensive to be explained by ordinary forgetfulness.

anhedonia. The inability to experience or even imagine any pleasant emotion.

anorexia. Loss of appetite.

anorgasmia. Inability to achieve orgasm.

anticipatory grief. A subjective state of emotional, physical, and social responses to an anticipated loss of a valued entity. The grief response is repeated once the loss actually occurs, but it may not be as intense as it might have been if anticipatory grieving had not occurred.

antisocial personality disorder. A pattern of socially irresponsible, exploitative, and guiltless behavior, evident in the tendency to fail to conform to the law, develop stable relationships, or sustain consistent employment; exploitation and manipulation of others for personal gain is common.

anxiety. Vague diffuse apprehension that is associated with feelings of uncertainty and helplessness.

associative looseness. Sometimes called loose associations, a thinking process characterized by speech in which ideas shift from one unrelated subject to another. The individual is unaware that the topics are unconnected.

ataxia. Muscular incoordination.

attitude. A frame of reference around which an individual organizes knowledge about his or her world. It includes an emotional element and can have a positive or negative connotation.

autism. A focus inward on a fantasy world and distorting or excluding the external environment; common in schizophrenia.

autistic disorder. The withdrawal of an infant or child into the self and into a fantasy world of his or her own creation. There is marked impairment in interpersonal functioning and communication and in imaginative play. Activities and interests are restricted and may be considered somewhat bizarre.

B

behavior modification. A treatment modality aimed at changing undesirable behaviors, using a system of reinforcement to bring about the modifications desired.

belief. An idea that one holds to be true. It can be rational, irrational, taken on faith, or stereotypical.

bereavement overload. An accumulation of grief that occurs when an individual experiences many losses over a short period and is unable to resolve one before another is experienced. This phenomenon is common among the elderly.

bipolar disorder. Characterized by mood swings from profound depression to extreme euphoria (mania), with intervening periods of normalcy. Psychotic symptoms may or may not be present.

borderline personality disorder. A disorder characterized by a pattern of intense and chaotic relationships, with affective instability, fluctuating and extreme attitudes regarding other people, impulsivity, direct and indirect self-destructive behavior, and lack of a clear or certain sense of identity, life plan, or values.

boundaries. The level of participation and interaction between individuals and between subsystems. Boundaries denote physical and psychological space individuals identify as their own. They are sometimes referred to as limits.

C

catatonia. A type of schizophrenia that is typified by stupor or excitement: stupor characterized by extreme psychomotor retardation, mutism, negativism, and posturing; excitement by psychomotor agitation, in which the movements are frenzied and purposeless.

circumstantiality. In speaking, the delay of an individual to reach the point of a communication owing to unnecessary and tedious details.

clang associations. A pattern of speech in which the choice of words is governed by sounds. Clang associations often take the form of rhyming.

codependency. An exaggerated dependent pattern of learned behaviors, beliefs, and feelings that make life painful. It is a dependence on people and things outside the self, along with neglect of the self to the point of having little self-identity.

cognition. Mental operations that relate to logic, awareness, intellect, memory, language, and reasoning powers.

cognitive therapy. A type of therapy in which the individual is taught to control thought distortions that are considered to be a factor in the development and maintenance of emotional disorders.

compensation. Covering up a real or perceived weakness by emphasizing a trait one considers more desirable.

concrete thinking. Thought processes that are focused on specifics rather than on generalities and immediate issues rather than eventual outcomes.

Individuals who are experiencing concrete thinking are unable to comprehend abstract terminology.

confidentiality. The right of an individual to the assurance that his or her case will not be discussed outside the boundaries of the health-care team.

crisis. Psychological disequilibrium in a person who confronts a hazardous circumstance that constitutes an important problem, which for the time he or she can neither escape nor solve with usual problem-solving resources.

crisis intervention. An emergency type of assistance in which the intervener becomes a part of the individual's life situation. The focus is to provide guidance and support to help mobilize the resources needed to resolve the crisis and restore or generate an improvement in previous level of functioning. Usually lasts no longer than 6 to 8 weeks.

culture. A particular society's entire way of living, encompassing shared patterns of belief, feeling, and knowledge that guide people's conduct and are passed down from generation to generation.

curandera. A female folk healer in the Latino culture.

curandero. A male folk healer in the Latino culture.

cycle of battering. Three phases of predictable behaviors that are repeated over time in a relationship between a batterer and a victim: the tension-building phase; the acute battering incident; and the calm, loving respite (honeymoon) phase.

cyclothymia. A chronic mood disturbance involving numerous episodes of hypomania and depressed mood, of insufficient severity or duration to meet the criteria for bipolar disorder.

D

delayed grief. Also called inhibited grief. The absence of evidence of grief when it ordinarily would be expected.

delirium. A state of mental confusion and excitement characterized by disorientation to time and place, often with hallucinations, incoherent speech, and a continual state of aimless physical activity.

delusions. False personal beliefs, not consistent with a person's intelligence or cultural background. The individual continues to have the belief in spite of obvious proof that it is false and/or irrational.

dementia. Global impairment of cognitive functioning that is progressive and interferes with social and occupational abilities.

denial. Refusal to acknowledge the existence of a real situation and/or the feelings associated with it.

depersonalization. An alteration in the perception or experience of the self so that the feeling of one's own reality is temporarily lost.

derealization. An alteration in the perception or experience of the external world so that it seems strange or unreal.

Diagnostic and Statistical Manual of Mental Disorders, 4th edition, Text Revision (DSM-IV-TR). Standard nomenclature of emotional illness published by the

American Psychiatric Association (APA) and used by all health-care practitioners. It classifies mental illness and presents guidelines and diagnostic criteria for various mental disorders.

displacement. Feelings are transferred from one target to another that is considered less threatening or neutral.

double-bind communication. Communication described as contradictory that places an individual in a "double bind." It occurs when a statement is made and succeeded by a contradictory statement or when a statement is made accompanied by nonverbal expression that is inconsistent with the verbal communication.

dyspareunia. Pain during sexual intercourse.

dysthymia. A depressive neurosis. The symptoms are similar to, if somewhat milder than, those ascribed to major depression. There is no loss of contact with reality.

dystonia. Involuntary muscular movements (spasms) of the face, arms, legs, and neck; may occur as an extrapyramidal side effect of some antipsychotic medications.

E

echolalia. The parrot-like repetition by an individual with loose ego boundaries of the words spoken by another.

ego. One of the three elements of the personality identified by Freud as the rational self, or "reality principle." The ego seeks to maintain harmony between the external world, the id, and the superego.

electroconvulsive therapy (ECT). A type of somatic treatment in which electric current is applied to the brain through electrodes placed on the temples. A grand mal seizure produces the desired effect. This is used with severely depressed patients refractory to antidepressant medications.

empathy. The ability to see beyond outward behavior and sense accurately another's inner experiencing. With empathy, one can accurately perceive and understand the meaning and relevance in the thoughts and feelings of another.

enmeshment. Exaggerated connectedness among family members. It occurs in response to diffuse boundaries in which there is overinvestment, overinvolvement, and lack of differentiation between individuals or subsystems.

ethnicity. The concept of people identifying with each other because of a shared heritage.

exhibitionism. A paraphilic disorder characterized by a recurrent urge to expose one's genitals to a stranger.

extrapyramidal symptoms (EPS). A variety of responses that originate outside the pyramidal tracts and in the basal ganglion of the brain. Symptoms may include tremors, chorea, dystonia, akinesia, and akathisia, and others may occur as a side effect of some antipsychotic medications.

F

family system. A system in which the parts of the whole may be the marital dyad, parent-child dyad, or sibling groups. Each of these subsystems is further divided into subsystems of individuals.

family therapy. A type of therapy in which the focus is on relationships within the family. The family is viewed as a system in which the members are interdependent, and a change in one creates change in all.

fight or flight. A syndrome of physical symptoms that result from an individual's real or perceived perception that harm or danger is imminent.

free association. A technique used to help individuals bring to consciousness material that has been repressed. The individual is encouraged to verbalize whatever comes into his or her mind, drifting naturally from one thought to another.

G

gains. The reinforcements an individual receives for somaticizing.

gender identity disorder. A sense of discomfort associated with an incongruence between biologically assigned gender and subjectively experienced gender.

generalized anxiety disorder. A disorder characterized by chronic (at least 6 months), unrealistic, and excessive anxiety and worry.

genogram. A graphic representation of a family system. It may cover several generations. Emphasis is on family roles and emotional relatedness among members. Genograms facilitate recognition of areas requiring change.

grief. A subjective state of emotional, physical, and social responses to the real or perceived loss of a valued entity. Change and failure can also be perceived as losses. The grief response consists of a set of relatively predictable behaviors that describe the subjective state that accompanies mourning.

group therapy. A therapy group, founded in a specific theoretical framework, led by a person with an advanced degree in psychology, social work, nursing, or medicine. The goal is to encourage improvement in interpersonal functioning.

H

hallucinations. False sensory perceptions not associated with real external stimuli. Hallucinations may involve any of the five senses.

histrionic personality disorder. Conscious or unconscious overly dramatic behavior used for drawing attention to oneself.

human immunodeficiency virus (HIV). The virus that is the etiological agent that produces the immunosuppression resulting in AIDS.

hypersomnia. Excessive sleepiness or seeking excessive amounts of sleep.

hypertensive crisis. A potentially life-threatening syndrome that results when an individual taking monoamine oxidase inhibitors (MAOIs) eats a product high in tyramine or uses a selective serotonin reuptake inhibitor too soon either before or after stopping an MAOI.

hypnosis. A treatment for disorders brought on by repressed anxiety. The individual is directed into a state of subconsciousness and assisted, through suggestions, to recall certain events that he or she cannot recall when conscious.

hypomania. A mild form of mania. Symptoms are excessive hyperactivity but not severe enough to cause marked impairment in social or occupational functioning or to require hospitalization.

I

id. One of the three components of the personality identified by Freud as the "pleasure principle." The id is the locus of instinctual drives, is present at birth, and compels the infant to satisfy needs and seek immediate gratification.

illusion. A misperception of a real external stimulus.

incest. Sexual exploitation of a child under 18 years of age by a relative or nonrelative who holds a position of trust in the family.

integration. The process used with individuals with dissociative identity disorder in an effort to bring all the personalities together into one; usually achieved through hypnosis.

intellectualization. An attempt to avoid expressing actual emotions associated with a stressful situation by using the intellectual processes of logic, reasoning, and analysis.

introjection. The beliefs and values of another individual are internalized and symbolically become a part of the self to the extent that the feeling of separateness or distinctness is lost.

isolation. The separation of a thought or a memory from the feeling, tone, or emotions associated with it (sometimes called emotional isolation).

J

justice. An ethical principle reflecting that all individuals should be treated equally and fairly.

K

kleptomania. A recurrent failure to resist impulses to steal objects not needed for personal use or monetary value.

Korsakoff's psychosis. A syndrome in alcoholics of confusion, loss of recent memory, and confabulation, caused by a deficiency of thiamine. It often occurs together with Wernicke's encephalopathy and may be termed Wernicke-Korsakoff syndrome.

L

libido. Freud's term for the psychic energy used to fulfill basic physiological needs or instinctual drives such as hunger, thirst, and sexuality.

limbic system. The part of the brain that is sometimes called the "emotional brain." It is associated with feelings of fear and anxiety; anger and aggression; love, joy, and hope; and with sexuality and social behavior.

long-term memory. Memory for remote events, or those that occurred many years ago. The type of memory that is preserved in the elderly individual.

loss. The experience of separation from something of personal importance.

luto. The word for mourning in the Mexican-American culture, which is symbolized by wearing black, black and white, or dark clothing and by subdued behavior.

M

magical thinking. A primitive form of thinking in which an individual believes that thinking about a possible occurrence can make it happen.

mania. A type of bipolar disorder in which the predominant mood is elevated, expansive, or irritable. Motor activity is frenzied and excessive. Psychotic features may or may not be present.

melancholia. A severe form of major depressive episode. Symptoms are exaggerated, and interest or pleasure in virtually all activities is lost.

mental imagery. A method of stress reduction that employs the imagination. The individual focuses imagination on a scenario that is particularly relaxing to him or her (e.g., a scene on a quiet seashore, a mountain atmosphere, or floating through the air on a fluffy white cloud).

milieu therapy. Also called therapeutic community, or therapeutic environment. This type of therapy consists of a scientific structuring of the environment in order to effect behavioral changes and to improve the individual's psychological health and functioning.

modeling. Learning new behaviors by imitating the behaviors of others.

mood. An individual's sustained emotional tone, which significantly influences behavior, personality, and perception.

mourning. The psychological process (or stages) through which the individual passes on the way to successful adaptation to the loss of a valued object.

N

narcissistic personality disorder. A disorder characterized by an exaggerated sense of self-worth. An individual lacks empathy and is hypersensitive to the evaluation of others.

neologism. New words a psychotic person invents that are meaningless to others but that have symbolic meaning to that individual.

neuroleptic. Antipsychotic medication used to prevent or control psychotic symptoms.

neuroleptic malignant syndrome (NMS). A rare but potentially fatal complication of treatment with neuroleptic drugs. Symptoms include severe muscle rigidity, high fever, tachycardia, fluctuations in blood pressure, diaphoresis, and rapid deterioration of mental status to stupor and coma.

neurotransmitter. A chemical that is stored in the axon terminals of the presynaptic neuron. An electrical impulse through the neuron stimulates the release of the neurotransmitter into the synaptic cleft, which in turn determines whether another electrical impulse is generated.

nursing diagnosis. A clinical judgment about individual, family, or community responses to actual and potential health problems/life processes. Nursing diagnoses provide the basis for selection of nursing interventions to achieve outcomes for which the nurse is accountable.

nursing process. A dynamic, systematic process by which nurses assess, diagnose, and identify outcomes; and plan, implement, and evaluate nursing care. It has been called "nursing's scientific methodology." Nursing process gives order and consistency to nursing intervention.

O

obesity. The state of having a body mass index of 30 or above.

object constancy. The phase in the separation/individuation process when the child learns to relate to objects in an effective, constant manner. A sense of separateness is established, and the child is able to internalize a sustained image of the loved object or person when out of sight.

obsessive-compulsive disorder. Recurrent thoughts or ideas (obsessions) that an individual is unable to put out of his or her mind, and actions that an individual is unable to refrain from performing (compulsions). The obsessions and compulsions are severe enough to interfere with social and occupational functioning.

oculogyric crisis. An attack of involuntary deviation and fixation of the eyeballs, usually in the upward position. It may last for several minutes or hours and may occur as an extrapyramidal side effect of some antipsychotic medications.

P

panic disorder. A disorder characterized by recurrent panic attacks, the onset of which is unpredictable and manifested by intense apprehension, fear, or terror, often associated with feelings of impending doom and accompanied by intense physical discomfort.

paranoia. A term that implies extreme suspiciousness. Paranoid schizophrenia is characterized by persecutory delusions and hallucinations of a threatening nature.

passive-aggressive behavior. Behavior that defends an individual's own basic rights by expressing resistance to social and occupational demands. Sometimes called indirect aggression, this behavior takes the form of sly, devious, and undermining actions that express the opposite of what the person is really feeling.

pedophilia. Recurrent urges and sexually arousing fantasies involving sexual activity with a prepubescent child.

perseveration. Persistent repetition of the same word or idea in response to different questions.

personality. Deeply ingrained patterns of behavior, which include the way one relates to, perceives, and thinks about the environment and oneself.

phobia. An irrational fear.

phobia, social. The fear of being humiliated in social situations.

postpartum depression. Depression that occurs during the postpartum period. It may be related to hormonal changes, tryptophan metabolism, or alterations in membrane transport during the early postpartum period. Other predisposing factors may also be influential.

posttraumatic stress disorder (PTSD). A syndrome of symptoms that develop following a psychologically distressing event that is outside the range of usual human experience (e.g., rape, war). The individual is unable to put the experience out of his or her mind and has nightmares, flashbacks, and panic attacks.

preassaultive tension state. Behaviors predictive of potential violence. They include excessive motor activity, tense posture, defiant affect, clenched teeth and fists, and other arguing, demanding, and threatening behaviors.

priapism. Prolonged painful penile erection; may occur as an adverse effect of some antidepressant medications, particularly trazodone.

progressive relaxation. A method of deep muscle relaxation in which each muscle group is alternately tensed and relaxed in a systematic order, with the person concentrating on the contrast of sensations experienced from tensing and relaxing.

projection. Attributing to another person feelings or impulses unacceptable to oneself.

pseudodementia. Symptoms of depression that mimic those of dementia.

psychomotor retardation. Extreme slowdown of physical movements. Posture slumps, speech is slowed, and digestion becomes sluggish. Common in severe depression.

psychotic disorder. A serious psychiatric disorder in which there is a gross disorganization of the personality, a marked disturbance in reality testing, and the impairment of interpersonal functioning and relationship to the external world.

R

rape. The expression of power and dominance by means of sexual violence, most commonly by men over women, although men may also be rape victims. Rape is considered an act of aggression, not of passion.

rapport. The development between two people in a relationship of special feelings based on mutual acceptance, warmth, friendliness, common interest, a sense of trust, and a nonjudgmental attitude.

rationalization. Attempting to make excuses or formulate logical reasons to justify unacceptable feelings or behaviors.

reaction formation. Preventing unacceptable or undesirable thoughts or behaviors from being expressed by exaggerating opposite thoughts or types of behaviors.

reframing. Changing the conceptual or emotional setting or viewpoint in relation to which a situation is experienced and placing it in another frame that fits the "facts" of the same concrete situation equally well or even better and thereby changing its entire meaning.

regression. A retreat to an earlier level of development and the comfort measures associated with that level of functioning.

reminiscence therapy. A process of life review by elderly individuals that promotes self-esteem and provides assistance in working through unresolved conflicts from the past.

repression. The involuntary blocking of unpleasant feelings and experiences from one's awareness.

ritualistic behavior. Purposeless activities that an individual performs repeatedly in an effort to decrease anxiety (e.g., hand washing); common in obsessive-compulsive disorder.

S

schizoid personality disorder. A profound defect in the ability to form personal relationships or to respond to others in any meaningful, emotional way.

schizotypal personality disorder. A disorder characterized by odd and eccentric behavior, not decompensating to the level of schizophrenia.

self-esteem. The amount of regard or respect that individuals have for themselves. It is a measure of worth that they place on their abilities and judgments.

shaman. The Native American "medicine man" or folk healer.

shaping. In learning, one shapes the behavior of another by giving reinforcements for increasingly closer approximations to the desired behavior.

short-term memory. The ability to remember events that occurred very recently. This ability deteriorates with age.

social skills training. Educational opportunities through role-play for the person with schizophrenia to learn appropriate social interaction skills and functional skills that are relevant to daily living.

splitting. A primitive ego defense mechanism in which the person is unable to integrate and accept both positive and negative feelings. In their view, people, including themselves, and life situations are all good or all bad. This trait is common in borderline personality disorder.

stereotyping. The process of classifying all individuals from the same culture or ethnic group as identical.

sublimation. The rechanneling of personally and/or socially unacceptable drives or impulses into activities that are tolerable and constructive.

substance abuse. Use of psychoactive drugs that poses significant hazards to health and interferes with social, occupational, psychological, or physical functioning.

substance dependence. Physical dependence is identified by the inability to stop using a substance despite attempts to do so; a continual use of the substance despite adverse consequences; a developing tolerance; and the development of withdrawal symptoms upon cessation or decreased intake. Psychological dependence is said to exist when a substance is perceived by the user to be necessary to maintain an optimal state of personal well-being, interpersonal relations, or skill performance.

substitution therapy. The use of various medications to decrease the intensity of symptoms in an individual who is withdrawing from, or experiencing the effects of excessive use of, substances.

superego. One of the three elements of the personality identified by Freud; represents the conscience and the culturally determined restrictions that are placed on an individual.

suppression. The voluntary blocking from one's awareness of unpleasant feelings and experiences.

symbiotic relationship. A type of "psychic fusion" that occurs between two people; it is unhealthy in that severe anxiety is generated in one or both if separation is indicated. A symbiotic relationship is normal between infant and mother.

sympathy. The actual sharing of another's thoughts and behaviors. Differs from empathy in that with empathy one experiences an objective understanding of what another is feeling rather than actually sharing those feelings.

systematic desensitization. A treatment for phobias in which the individual is taught to relax and then asked to imagine various components of the phobic stimulus on a graded hierarchy, moving from that which produces the least fear to that which produces the most.

T

tangentiality. The inability to get to the point of a story. The speaker introduces many unrelated topics until the original topic of discussion is lost.

tardive dyskinesia. Syndrome of symptoms characterized by bizarre facial and tongue movements, a stiff neck, and difficulty swallowing. It may occur as an adverse effect of long-term therapy with some antipsychotic medications.

thought-stopping technique. A self-taught technique that an individual uses each time he or she wishes to eliminate intrusive or negative unwanted thoughts from awareness.

triangles. A three-person emotional configuration that is considered the basic building block of the family system. When anxiety becomes too great between two family members, a third person is brought in to form a triangle. Triangles are dysfunctional in that they offer relief from anxiety through diversion rather than through resolution of the issue.

trichotillomania. The recurrent failure to resist impulses to pull out one's own hair.

tyramine. An amino acid found in aged cheeses or other aged, overripe, and fermented foods; broad beans; pickled herring; beef or chicken liver; preserved meats; beer and wine; yeast products; chocolate; caffeinated drinks; canned figs; sour cream; yogurt; soy sauce; and some over-the-counter cold medications and diet pills. If foods high in tyramine content are consumed when an individual is taking MAOIs, a potentially life-threatening syndrome called hypertensive crisis can result.

U

unconditional positive regard. Carl Rogers' term for the respect and dignity of an individual regardless of his or her unacceptable behavior.

undoing. A mechanism used to symbolically negate or cancel out a previous action or experience that one finds intolerable.

universality. One curative factor of groups (identified by Yalom) in which individuals realize that they are not alone in a problem and in the thoughts and feelings they are experiencing. Anxiety is relieved by the support and understanding of others in the group who share similar experiences.

V

values. Personal beliefs about the truth, beauty, or worth of a thought, object, or behavior that influences an individual's actions.

velorio. In the Mexican-American culture, large numbers of family and friends gather following a death for a festive watch over the body of the deceased person before burial.

W

Wernicke's encephalopathy. A brain disorder caused by thiamine deficiency and characterized by visual disturbances, ataxia, somnolence, stupor, and, without thiamine replacement, death.

word salad. A group of words that are put together in a random fashion without any logical connection.

Pregnancy Categories

Category A

Adequate, well-controlled studies in pregnant women have not shown an increased risk of fetal abnormalities.

Category B

Animal studies have revealed no evidence of harm to the fetus, however, there are no adequate and well-controlled studies in pregnant women.

OR

Animal studies have shown an adverse effect, but adequate and well-controlled studies in pregnant women have failed to demonstrate a risk to the fetus.

Category C

Animal studies have shown an adverse effect and there are no adequate and well-controlled studies in pregnant women.

OR

No animal studies have been conducted and there are no adequate and well-controlled studies in pregnant women.

Category D

Studies, adequate well-controlled or observational, in pregnant women have demonstrated a risk to the fetus. However, the benefits of therapy may outweigh the potential risk.

Category X

Studies, adequate well-controlled or observational, in animals or pregnant women have demonstrated positive evidence of fetal abnormalities. The use of the product is contraindicated in women who are or may become pregnant.

NOTE: The designation UK is used when the pregnancy category is unknown.

References

American Hospital Association. A Patient's Bill of Rights (revised 1992)

American Hospital Association. A Patient Care Partnership (2003). Accessed 12/19/10 at: http://www.aha.org/aha/issues/Communicating-With-Patients/pt-care-partnership.html

American Psychiatric Association. Diagnostic and Statistical Manual of Mental Disorders, 4th ed., Text Revision. Washington, DC: American Psychiatric Association, 2000

American Psychiatric Association. Position Statement: Principles for Health Care Reform in Psychiatry, 2008

American Psychiatric Nurses Association (APNA). Seclusion and Restraint: Position Statement & Standards of Practice, 2007

Andersson M, Zetterberg H, Minthon L, Blennow K, Londos E. The cognitive profile and CSF biomarkers in dementia with Lewy bodies and Parkinson's disease dementia. Int J Geriatr Psychiatry 2011; Jan 26(1):100–105

Anton RF et al. Comparison of bio-rad %CDT TIA and CD Tect as laboratory markers of heavy alcohol use and their relationships with γ-glutamyl-transferase. Clinical Chemistry 2001; 47:1769–1775

APA 2000 Gender Advisory Panel: Terms of Reference. Accessed 7/17/04 at: www.who.int/reproductive-health/pcc2001/documents/gaptorrev01.doc

Arana GW, Rosenbaum JF. Handbook of Psychiatric Drug Therapy, 5th ed. Philadelphia: Lippincott Williams & Wilkins, 2005

Aripiprazole (Abilify). Accessed 1/4/11 at: http://www.abilify.com

Asenapine (Saphris). Accessed 1/5/11 at: http://www.saphris.com

Autonomic nervous system. Table 1: Responses of major organs to autonomic nerve impulses. Update in Anaesthesia 1995; issue 5, article 6. Accessed 1/24/04 at: http://www.nda.ox.ac.uk/wfsa/html/u05/u05_b02.htm

Barr AM et al. The need for speed: An update on methamphetamine addiction. Psychiatr Neurosci 2006; 31(5):301–313

Bateson G. Steps to an Ecology of Mind. London: Paladin, 1973

Bateson G. Mind and Nature: A Necessary Unity. London: Wildwood House, 1979

Bleuler E. Dementia Praecox or the Group of Schizophrenias (Zinkin J, trans.). New York: International University Press, 1911

Boszormenyi-Nagy I, Krasner BR. Between Give and Take: A Clinical Guide to Contextual Therapy. New York: Brunner/Mazel, 1986

Bowen M. Family Therapy in Clinical Practice. New Jersey: Aronson, 1994

Brigham and Women's Hospital. Depression: A Guide to Diagnosis and Treatment. Boston, MA: Brigham and Women's Hospital, 2001:9

Brown AS, Susser ES. Epidemiology of schizophrenia: Findings implicate neurodevelopmental insults early in life. In: Kaufman CA, Gorman JM, eds. Schizophrenia: New Directions for Clinical Research and Treatment. Larchmont, NY: Mary Ann Liebert, Inc., 1996:105–119

Brown GW, Birley JL, Wing JK. Influence of family life on the course of schizophrenic disorders: A replication. Br J Psychiatry 1972; 121(562):241–258

Burgess AW, Hartman CR. Rape trauma and posttraumatic stress disorder. In: McBride AB, Austin JK, eds. Psychiatric Mental Health Nursing: Integrating the Behavioral and Biological Sciences. Philadelphia: WB Saunders, 1996:53–81

Buse JB et al. A retrospective cohort study of diabetes mellitus and antipsychotic treatment in the United States. J Clin Epidemiol 2003; 56:164–170

Chenitz WC, Stone JT, Salisbury SA. Clinical Gerontological Nursing: A Guide to Advanced Practice. Philadelphia: WB Saunders, 1991

Child Abuse Prevention Treatment Act, originally enacted in 1974 (PL 93–247), 42 USC 5101 et seq; 42 USC 5116 et seq. Accessed 9/25/04 at: http://www. acf.hhs.gov/programs/cb/laws/capta/

Christianson JR, Blake RH. The grooming process in father-daughter incest. In: Horton A, Johnson BL, Roundy LM, Williams D, eds. The Incest Perpetrator: A Family Member No One Wants to Treat. Newbury Park, CA: Sage, 1990:88–98

Christy A, Handelsman JB, Hanson A, Ochshorn E. Who initiates emergency commitments? Community Ment Health J 2010; Apr 46(2): 188–191

Combs DR, Waguspack J, Chapman D et al. An examination of social cognition, neurocognition, and symptoms as predictors of social functioning in schizophrenia. Schizophr Res 2010; Dec 13 [Epub]

Cruz M, Pincus HA. Research on the influence that communication in psychiatric encounters has on treatment. Psychiatr Serv 2002; 53:1253–1265

Cyberonics (2007). Accessed 1/3/11 at: http://www.VNSTherapy.com

Cycle of Violence. Accessed 8/7/04 at: http://www.ojp.usdoj.gov/ovc/help/cycle.htm

Davies T. Psychosocial factors and relapse of schizophrenia [editorial]. BMJ 1994; 309:353–354

DeAngelis T. Is Internet addiction real? Monitor on Psychology. American Psychological Association 2000; 31: No. 4. Accessed 11/27/2006 at: www.apa.org/monitor/apr00/addiction.html

DSM-V: Introduction to dimensional assessments. Medscape: Psychology and wellbeing. May 27, 2009. Accessed 12/23/10 at: http://www.psychologyandwellbeing.org/pn/ modules.php?name=News&file=article&sid=162

DSM-5.org. Accessed 1/3/10 at: http://www.dsm5.org/Pages/Default.aspx

Edmondson OJH, Psychogiou L, Vlachos H et al. Depression in fathers in the postnatal period: Assessment of the Edinburgh Postnatal Depression Scale as a screening measure. J Affect Disord 2010; Sept 125(1-3):365–368

Emergency Commitments: Psychiatric emergencies. Accessed 1/24/04 at: http://www.pinofpa.org/resources/fact-12.html

European College of Neuropsychopharmacology Congress (ECNP): Zyprexa (olanzapine) superior to depakote (Valproate) for acute mania in bipolar disorder. Accessed 11/29/2006 at: http://www.pslgroup.com/dg/1E0626.htm

Ewing JA. Detecting alcoholism: The CAGE Questionnaire. JAMA 1984; 252:1905–1907

Faraone S. Prevalence of adult ADHD in the US [abstract]. Presented at American Psychiatric Association, May 6, 2004. Accessed 9/24/04 at: http://www.pslgroup.com/dg/2441a2.htm

Folstein M, Folstein SG, McHugh P. Mini-Mental State, a practical method for grading the cognitive state of patients for the clinician. J Psychiatr Res 1975; 12:189–198

Fox S. DSM-V, Healthcare reform will fuel major changes in addiction psychiatry. Medscape medical news 2010. Accessed 12/23/10 at: http://www.medscape.com/viewarticle/733649

Frances A. A warning sign on the road to DSM-V: Beware of its unintended consequences. Psychiatric Times 2009; 26(8): June 26. Accessed 12/23/10 at http://www.psychiatrictimes.com

Frazer A, Molinoff P, Winokur A. Biological Bases of Brain Function and Disease. New York: Raven Press, 1994

Freeman A et al. Clinical Applications of Cognitive Therapy, 2nd ed. New York: Springer Verlag, 2004

Fruchtnict S. The DSM-5 controversy. Brooklyn Health News Examiner. May 3, 2010

Fuller MA, Sajatovic M: Drug Information Handbook for Psychiatry: Including Psychotropic, Non-Psychotropic, and Herbal Agents, 7th ed. Cleveland: Lexi-Comp, 2009

George MS, Lisanby SH, Avery D et al. Daily left prefrontal transcranial magnetic stimulation therapy for major depressive disorder. Arch Gen Psychiatry 2010; 67(5):507–516

Ghaemi SN et al. Antidepressants in bipolar disorder: The case for caution. Bipolar Disord 2003; 5:421–433

Goroll AH, Mulley AG Jr. Primary Care Medicine: Office Evaluation and Management of the Adult Patient, 6th ed. Philadelphia: Lippincott Williams & Wilkins, 2009

Guy W, ed. ECDEU Assessment Manual for Psychopharmacology. (DHEW Publ. No. 76–338), rev. ed. Washington, DC: US Department of Health, Education and Welfare, 1976

Health Canada: Important drug safety information for paroxetine. Accessed 9/25/04 at: http://www.hc-sc.gc.ca/hpfb-dgpsa/tpd-dpt/paxil_hpc_e.html

Health Insurance Portability and Accountability Act (HIPAA). Accessed 11/27/06 at: http://www.ihs.gov/AdminMngrResources/HIPAA/index.cfm

Hernandez AE. Global Symposium: Examining the relationship between online and offline offenses and preventing the sexual exploitation of children, April 5-7, 2009. Accessed Dec 29, 2010 at: http://www.iprc.unc.edu/G8/Hernandez_position_paper_Global_Symposium.pdf

Hirschfeld RM, Williams JB, Spitzer RL et al. Development and validation of a screening instrument for bipolar spectrum disorder: The Mood Disorder Questionnaire. Am J Psychiatry 2000; 157:1873–1875

Hirschfeld RMA, Holzer C, Calabrese JR, Weissman M, Reed M, Davies M, Frye MA, Keck P et al. Validity of the Mood Disorder Questionnaire: A general population study. Am J Psychiatry 2003; 160:178–180

Holkup P. Evidence-based protocol: Elderly suicide: Secondary prevention. Iowa City: University of Iowa Gerontological Nursing Interventions Research Center, Research Dissemination Core, June 2002:56

Holtzheimer PE, Nemeroff CB. Advances in the treatment of depression. NeuroRx 2006; 3:42–56

Hunt M. The Story of Psychology. New York: Anchor Books, 1994

Iloperidone (Fanapt). Accessed 1/5/11 at: http://www.fanapt.com

International Society of Psychiatric–Mental Health Nurses (ISPN). ISPN Position statement on the use of seclusion and restraint (November 1999). Accessed 11/27/06 at: http://www.ispn-psych.org

Jahoda M. Current Concepts of Positive Mental Health. New York: Basic Books, 1958

Johnson TB. National Association of School Psychologists Communiqué. October 2003; vol. 32, No. 2. Accessed 9/25/04 at: http://www.nasponline.org/publications/cq322depressionwarnings.html

Joint Commission on Accreditation of Healthcare Organizations (JCAHO 2005). Restraint and Seclusion, revised April 1, 2005. Accessed 11/25/06 at: http://www.jcaho.org/

Kansas Child Abuse Prevention Council (KCAPC). A Guide about Child Abuse and Neglect. Wichita, KS: National Committee for Prevention of Child Abuse and Parents Anonymous, 1992

Keck PE Jr. Evaluating treatment decisions in bipolar depression. MedScape July 30, 2003. Accessed 7/3/04 at: http:www. medscape.com/viewpro-gram/2571

Keltner NL, Folks DG. Psychotropic Drugs, 4th ed. St. Louis: Mosby-Year Book, 2005

Kerr ME, Bowen M. Family Evaluation. New York: WW Norton, 1988

Krupnick SLW. Psychopharmacology. In Lego S (ed). Psychiatric Nursing: A Comprehensive Reference, 2nd ed. Philadelphia: Lippincott-Raven, 1996:499–541

Kübler-Ross E. On Death and Dying. New York: Touchstone, 1997

Kukull WA, Bowen JD. Dementia epidemiology. Med Clin North Am 2002; 86:3

Lego S. Psychiatric Nursing. A Comprehensive Reference, 2nd ed. Philadelphia: Lippincott-Raven 1996

Linehan MM. Cognitive-Behavioral Treatment of Borderline Personality Disorder. New York: Guilford Press, 1993

Lippitt R, White RK. An experimental study of leadership and group life. In Maccoby EE, Newcomb TM, Hartley EL, eds. Readings in Social Psychology, 3rd ed. New York: Holt Rinehart & Winston, 1958

Lubman DI, Castle DJ. Late-onset schizophrenia: Make the right diagnosis when psychosis emerges after age 60. Curr Psychiatry Online 2002; 1(12).

Accessed 8/7/04 at: http://www.currentpsychiatry.com/2002_12/1202_schizo.asp

Lurasidone (Latuda). Accessed 1/5/11 at: http://www.latuda.com

Major Theories of Family Therapy. Accessed 8/2/04 at: http://www.goldentriadfilms.com/films/theory.htm

Manos PJ. 10-point clock test screens for cognitive impairment in clinic and hospital settings. Psychiatric Times 1998; 15(10). Accessed 9/20/04 at: http://www.psychiatrictimes.com/p981049.html

Maxmen JS, Kennedy SH, McIntyre RS. Psychotropic Drugs Fast Facts, 4th ed. New York: WW Norton, 2008

Mayo Clinic. Mayo Clinic study using structural MRI may help accurately diagnose dementia patients (July 11, 2009). Accessed 12/20/10 at: http://www.mayoclinic.org/news2009-rst/5348.html

McGoldrick M, Giordano J, Garcia-Preto N. Ethnicity and Family Therapy, 3rd ed. New York: Guilford Press, 2005

Melrose S. Paternal postpartum depression: How can nurses begin to help? Contemp Nurse 2010 Feb-Mar; 34(2):199–210

Meltzer HY, Baldessarini RJ. Reducing the risk for suicide in schizophrenia and affective disorders: Academic highlights. J Clin Psychiatry 2003; 64:9

Mentalhealthcarereform.org. Accessed 12/19/10

Mini-Mental State Examination form. Available from Psychological Assessment Resources, Inc., 16204 North Florida Ave, Lutz, Florida (see http://www.parinc.com/index.cfm)

M'Naughton Rule. Psychiatric News 2002; 37(8)

Murray RB, Zentner JP. Health Assessment and Promotion Strategies through the Life Span, 6th ed. Stamford, CT: Appleton & Lange, 1997

Myers E. LPNotes: Nurses Clinical Pocket Guide, 2nd ed. Philadelphia: FA Davis, 2007

Myers E. RNotes: Nurses Clinical Pocket Guide, 3rd ed. Philadelphia: FA Davis, 2010

Nagy Ledger of Merits. Accessed 8/2/04 at: http://www. behavenet.com/capsules/treatment/famsys/ldgermrts.htm

National Institutes of Health (US). Grady C. Informed consent: The ideal and the reality, Session 5. Aired November 9, 2005; permanent link: http://videocast.nih.gov/Summary.asp?File=12895. Accessed 12/19/10

National Institute of Mental Health (NIMH). The numbers count: Mental disorders in America. Accessed 12/26/10 at: http://www.nimh.nih.gov/

health/publications/the-numbers-count-mental-disorders-in-america/index.shtml

Neilsen J, Skadhede S, Correll CU. Antipsychotics associated with the development of type 2 diabetes in antipsychotic-naïve schizophrenia patients. Neuropsychopharmacology 2010; 35: Aug 2010

Nelson JC, Mankoski R, Baker RA. Effects of aripiprazole adjunctive to standard antidepressant treatment on the core symptoms of depression: A post-hoc, pooled analysis of two large, placebo-controlled studies. 2010-01, J Affect Disord 120(1-3):133–140.

Nemeroff CB et al. VNS therapy in treatment-resistant depression: Clinical evidence and putative neurobiological mechanisms. Neuropsychopharmacology 2006; 31:1345–1355

Ng BD, Wiemer-Hastings P. Addiction to the Internet and online gaming. Cyberpsychol Behav 2005; 8:110–113

Nonacs RM. Postpartum depression. eMedicine June 17, 2004. Accessed 7/17/04 at: http://www.emedicine.com/med/topic3408.html

Olanzapine + VA, Lithium vs Valproic Acid, Lithium: Therapeutic use: Bipolar disorders Accessed 8/1/04 at: http://www.luinst. org/cp/en/CNSforum/literature/trial_reports/reports/889317.html

Paliperidone (Invega). Product insert/prescribing information. Issued December 2006, Janssen, LP. Accessed 12/29/06 at: http://www.invega.com

Paquette M. Managing anger effectively. Accessed 8/2/04 at: http://www.nurseweek.com/ce/ce290a.html

Patient's Bill of Rights: American Hospital Association. Accessed 1/18/04 at: http://joann980.tripod.com/myhomeontheweb/id20.html

Pedersen D. Pocket Psych Drugs: Point-of-care clinical guide. Philadelphia: FA Davis, 2010

Peplau H. A working definition of anxiety. In: Bird S, Marshall M, eds. Some Clinical Approaches to Psychiatric Nursing. New York: Macmillan, 1963

Peplau HE. Interpersonal Relations in Nursing. New York: Springer, 1992

Poulin C, Webster I, Single E. Alcohol disorders in Canada as indicated by the CAGE Questionnaire. Can Med Assoc J 1997; 157:1529–1535

Purnell LD. Guide to Culturally Competent Health Care, 2nd ed. Philadelphia: FA Davis, 2009

Purnell LD, Paulanka BJ. Transcultural Health Care: A Culturally Competent Approach, 3rd ed. Philadelphia: FA Davis

Quality and Safety Education for Nurses (QSEN). Accessed 1/15/11 at: http://www.qsen.org

Rachid F, Bertschy G. Safety and efficacy of repetitive transcranial magnetic stimulation in the treatment of depression: A critical appraisal of the last 10 years. Neurophysiol Clin 2006; 36:157–183

Rakel R. Saunders Manual of Medical Practice, 2nd ed. Philadelphia: WB Saunders, 2000

Ramelteon (Rozerem): Prescribing information. Accessed 1/3/11 at: http://www.rozerem.com/en/?

Reiger DA et al. Comorbidity of mental disorders with alcohol and other drug abuse. JAMA 1990; 246:2511–2518

Reno J. Domestic Violence Awareness. Office of the Attorney General. Accessed 9/25/04 at: http://www.ojp.usdoj.gov/ovc/help/cycle.htm (last updated 4/19/2001)

Rosner S, Hackl-Herrwerth A, Leucht S, Vecchi S, Sisurapanont M, Soyka M. Opioid antagonists for alcohol dependence. Cochrane Database Syst Rev. 2010; Dec 8:12

Rupp A, Keith SJ. The costs of schizophrenia: Assessing the burden. Psychiatr Clin North Am 1993; 16:413–423

Sadock BJ, Sadock VA, Ruiz P. Kaplan & Sadock's Comprehensive Textbook of Psychiatry, 9th ed. Baltimore: Lippincott Williams & Wilkins, 2009

Satcher D. Mental Health: A Report of the Surgeon General. Rockville, MD: US Department of Health and Human Services, Substance Abuse and Mental Health Services Administration, Center for Mental Health Services, National Institutes of Health, National Institute of Mental Health, 1999. Accessed 1/19/04 at: http://www.surgeongeneral.gov/library/mentalhealth/home.html

Scanlon VC, Sanders T. Essentials of Anatomy and Physiology, 5th ed. Philadelphia: FA Davis, 2007

Schloendorff v. Society of New York Hospital, 105 NE 92 (NY 1914)

Schwarz E, Izmailov R, Spain M. Validation of a blood-based laboratory test to aid in the confirmation of a diagnosis of schizophrenia. Biomarker Insights 2010; 5:39–47

Science News (Jan 17, 2008). Post traumatic stress tripled among combat-exposed military personnel. Accessed 1/3/11 at: http://www.sciencedaily.com/releases/2008/01/080116193412.htm

Segal ZV, Bieling P, Young T et al. Antidepressant monotherapy vs sequential pharmacotherapy and mindfulness-based cognitive therapy, or placebo, for relapse prophylaxis in recurrent depression. Arch Gen Psychiartry 2010; 67(12):1256–1264

Selegiline Transdermal System (Emsam) Prescribing information. Accessed 1/3/11 at: http://www.emsam.com/

Selye H. The Stress of Life. New York: McGraw-Hill, 1976

Selzer ML, Vinokur A, van Rooijen L. A self-administered Short Michigan Alcoholism Screening Test (SMAST). J Stud Alcohol 1975; 36:117–126

Shapiro F. Eye Movement Desensitization and Reprocessing: Basic Principles, Protocols, and Procedures, 2nd ed. New York: Guilford Press, 2001

Shea CA et al. American Psychiatric Nurses Association. Advanced Practice Nursing in Psychiatric and Mental Health Care. St. Louis: CV Mosby, 1999

Sheikh JI, Yesavage JA. Geriatric Depression Scale (GDS): Recent evidence and development of a shorter version. In: Brink TL, ed. Clinical Gerontology: A Guide to Assessment and Intervention. New York: Haworth Press, 1986:165–173

Skinner K. The therapeutic milieu: Making it work. J Psychiatr Nursing Mental Health Serv 1979; 17:38–44

Smith GR, Kramer TL, Hollenberg JA et al. Validity of the Depression-Arkansas (D-ARK) scale: A tool for measuring major depressive disorder. Mental Health Services Research 2002; 4

Smith M, Hopkins D, Peveler RC et al. First- v. second-generation antipsychotics and risk for diabetes in schizophrenia: Systematic review and meta-analysis. Br J Psychiatry 2008; Jun 192(6):406–411

Sonne SC, Brady KT. Bipolar Disorder and Alcoholism. National Institute on Alcohol Abuse and Alcoholism (NIAAA). Posted November 2002. Accessed 7/3/04 at: http://www.niaaa.nih.gov/publications/arh26–2/103–108.htm

Stiles MM, Koren C, Walsh K. Identifying elder abuse in the primary care setting. Clin Geriatr 2002; 10. Accessed 8/7/04 at: http://www.mmhc.com

Stuart MR, Lieberman JA. The Fifteen-Minute Hour: Therapeutic Talk in Primary Care. Oxford: Radcliffe Publishing, 2008

Suicide Risk Factors. Accessed 8/7/04 at: http://www.infoline.org/crisis/ risk.asp

Susser E, Schwartz S, Morabia A, Bromet, E. Psychiatric Epidemiology: Searching for the Causes of Mental Disorders. New York: Oxford University Press, 2006

Tai B, Blaine J. Naltrexone: An Antagonist Therapy for Heroin Addiction. Presented at the National Institute on Drug Abuse, November 12–13, 1997. Accessed 7/3/2004 at: http://www.nida.nih.gov/MeetSum/naltrexone.html

Tarasoff v. Regents of University of California (17 Cal. 3d 425 – July 1, 1976. S. F. No. 23042)

Townsend MC. Essentials of Psychiatric Mental Health Nursing: Concepts of Care in Evidence Based Practice, 5th ed. Philadelphia: FA Davis, 2010

Townsend MC. Psychiatric Mental Health Nursing: Concepts of Care in Evidence-Based Practice, 6th ed. Philadelphia: FA Davis, 2009

Travelbee J. Interpersonal Aspects of Nursing. Philadelphia: FA Davis, 1971

Tucker K. Milan Approach to Family Therapy: A Critique. Accessed 8/2/04 at: http://www.priory.com/psych/milan.htm

US Department of Health and Human Services: HIPAA. Accessed 11/27/2006

US Food and Drug Administration (FDA). Antidepressant Use in Children, Adolescents and Adults. Accessed 5/10/07 at: www.fda.gov/cder/drug/antidepressants/default.htm

US Food and Drug Administration (FDA). FDA Requests Label Change for All Sleep Disorder Drug Products. Accessed 5/11/07 at: www.fda.gov/bbs/topics/NEWS/2007/NEW01587.html

US Public Health Services (USPHS). The Surgeon General's Call to Action to Prevent Suicide. Washington, DC: US Department of Health and Human Services, 1999. Accessed 1/18/04 at: http://www.surgeongeneral.gov/library/calltoaction/calltoaction.htm

Vallerand AH, Sanoski CA, Deglin JH. Davis's Drug Guide for Nurses, 12th ed. Philadelphia: FA Davis, 2011

Van der Kolk BA. Trauma and memory. In: Van der Kolk BA, McFarlane AC, Weisaeth L. Traumatic Stress. New York: Guilford Press, 1996

Van Leeuwen AM, Poelhuis-Leth DJ, Bladh ML. Davis's Comprehensive Handbook of Laboratory and Diagnostic Tests with Nursing Implications, 4th ed. Philadelphia: FA Davis, 2011

VeriPsych Biomarker Blood Test. Accessed 12/24/10 at: http://www.veripsych.com/physician-faq

Vermuri P, Jack CR Jr. Role of structural MRI in Alzheimer's disease. Alzheimer's Res Ther 2010; Aug 31 2(4):23

Virginia S. In Allyn & Bacon Family Therapy Web Site. Accessed 8/2/04 at: http://www.abacon.com/famtherapy/satir.html

Walker LE. The Battered Woman. New York: Harper & Row, 1979

Walter LJ et al. The Depression-Arkansas scale: A validation study of a new brief depression scale in an HMO. J Clin Psychol 2003; 59:465–481

Weathers FW, Huska JA, Keane TM. PCL-C for DSM-IV. Boston: National Center for PTSD–Behavioral Science Division, 1991.

WebMD Video: Caregiver Stress. Accessed 12/20/10 at: http://www.webmd.com/video/caregiving-stress

World Health Organization (WHO) (1975, 2002). Sexual Health and Sex. Accessed 11/27/06 at: http://www.who.int/reproductive-health/gender/sexual_health.html

Yalom ID, Leszcz M. The Theory and Practice of Group Psychotherapy, 5th ed. New York: Perseus Books, 2005

Yesavage JA et al. Development and validation of a geriatric depression screening scale: A preliminary report. J Psychiatr Res 1983; 17:37–49

Young People Advised Not to Use Seroxat. 10 Downing Street, Newsroom, October 6, 2003. Accessed 9/25/04 at: http://www.number-10.gov.uk/output/page3851.asp

Zyprexa (Eli Lilly Company). Accessed 1/3/11 at: http://pi.lilly. com/us/zyprexa-pi.pdf

Credits

Dosage and drug data in Psychotropic Drug Tab from Table 17.6, p. 466 (Antianxiety Agents); Table 15.3, p. 383 (Antidepressants), Table 16.6, p. 419 (Mood Stabilizing Agents), and Table 14.5, p. 342 (Antipsychotics), in Townsend MC. Essentials of Psychiatric Mental Health Nursing, 5th ed., 2011, and from Deglin JH, Vallerand AH, Sanoski CA. Davis's Drug Guide for Nurses, 12th ed. Philadelphia: FA Davis, 2011, and Pedersen: Pocket Psych Drugs, Philadelphia, FA Davis, 2010, with permission.

DSM-IV-TR criteria in Disorders tab, Global Assessment of Functioning (GAF) form, Multiaxial System, and DSM-IV-TR classifications: Axes I and II categories and codes, reprinted with permission from the Diagnostic and Statistical Manual of Mental Disorders, 4th ed., Text Revision. Washington, DC: American Psychiatric Association, 2000.

Index

Note: Page numbers followed by f refer to figures/illustrations.

D

M

N